"Give Me 90 Days And I GUARANTEE To Completely RESHAPE Your Body!"

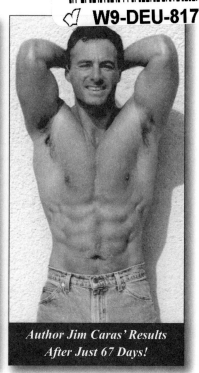

Author Jim Caras Before Using This System…

Author Jim Caras' Results After Just 67 Days!

"Isn't it comforting to know that after all you have, (or haven't done) to your body in the last 5-10 years, you can completely change your body in less than 90 days – and for the rest of your life?

Jim Caras
Author

All photos in this book are actual, untouched photos of the author, Jim Caras and his readers. Contrary to what most people assume, Jim and his readers transformed their bodies by eating 4-5 healthy meals a day, without being hungry, and with minimal exercise – on average, 45 minutes, three days a week.

How to Completely
RESHAPE
YOUR BODY!™

**A Proven, Step-By-Step Guide To
Losing Weight and Shaping Your Body**

By Jim Caras

Note To The Reader And Legal Notices:

This publication contains the opinions and ideas of its author. It is intended to provide helpful and informative material on the subjects addressed in the publication. It is sold with the understanding that the author and publisher are not engaged in rendering medical, health, or any other kind of personal professional services in the book. The reader should consult his or her medical, health, or other competent professional before adopting any of the suggestions in this book or drawing inferences from it.

This publication is for informational purposes only and should not be used as a guide for diagnosis and treatment of any disease. If you have health problems, you should seek the advice of a health care professional. The author and publisher disclaim all responsibility for any liability, loss, injury or damage incurred as a consequence directly or indirectly of the use and application of any of the contents herein.

The eating plans presented here are not intended or designed for anyone with kidney problems or for pregnant women, nursing mothers or women who are trying to get pregnant. If you are on any medication or have cholesterol problems, high blood pressure, diabetes, an abnormal heart rhythm or any cardiovascular disease, have had a heart attack, or have any known heart problems – do not under any circumstances attempt or begin this program without a physician's guidance and close supervision. Even readers not subject to any of the above problems or medical limitations should consult a physician before beginning this or any diet, supplement or fitness program.

Table of Contents

Thank <u>you</u> for inspiring me...

I dedicate this book to all those brave and inspiring people who seek to conquer their physical limitations, so they can fulfill their true life purpose, while improving their lives and all those around them.

I also dedicate this book to my mother who has always stood beside me, believed in me, encouraged me – and lent me $1,500 when I had nothing, to print the original version of this book and develop the Health Direct products that have improved the lives of over 1 million people over the last 10 years.

"Why This Is One Of The Most Authentic Books On Weight Loss You'll Ever Read..."

There are many books on weight loss, and more coming out, seemingly every day. With Americans becoming increasingly overweight, many nutritional companies, medical professionals, pharmaceutical companies, and opportunists, recognize it as a way to make a quick buck – and for some – massive amounts of money. The resulting weight loss supplements, dangerous metabolic stimulants and drugs, and books with fancy or impressive sounding titles have flooded the market to lure those of us who battle with our weight.

This was never the case with this book.

The Problem With Most Other Weight Loss Books And Authors...

Unlike most of the other weight loss authors, I have battled with my weight (even as a child), just like you. Also, unlike most weight loss authors, everything in the book was developed and used by me to lose weight, reshape my body, and improve my health.

The problem I personally have with most other programs and books is that they are written by people who have *not* battled their weight like you and I have. The problem is...

They Don't Know What It Is Like To Be Overweight...

Most of the people who write weight loss books – naturally thin people, doctors, fitness gurus, celebrities. – really don't know what it is like to be overweight and to struggle to lose weight. Don't get me wrong, there is some really good information, research, and concepts out there. BUT unless the author actually has been overweight and done the program themselves, they really don't understand what is going through our minds and how to structure their programs to overcome the thoughts, beliefs, and temptations that challenge us.

What they don't know and can't learn from research, facts, or putting other people or patients on their program is what its like to:

- Stand there in the morning, or before going out to a social event, stare aimlessly in your closet for clothing that makes you look the least fat.

- Struggle to button or zip up your clothes.

- Go shopping and be horrified when seeing your bulging fat in the mirror of the dressing room. Do you ever wonder if the stores buy the left-over mirrors from the fun house at the circus?

- Feel depressed during the day or at that special event when your clothing is tight and you feel fat.

- Have naturally thin people and doctors tell you to "eat less" and/or "exercise more" – especially when it's not working.

- Be hungry all the time; to never have that satisfied feeling when eating that makes you want to stop.

- Crave sweets and caffeinated beverages.

- Crave sweets at night, even after you've eaten a satisfying meal.

- Buy new clothes, and not only be discouraged at your "new" larger size, but being embarrassed to tell the store clerk what size you are (as you sheepishly say, "I'm usually a 4, but some clothes fit me as an 8," when you're actually an 8).

- Avoid outdoor events (beaches, lakes, etc.) or special events (like reunions) because of how you look.

I can go on and on - and only those of us who have been there know what I am talking about - they can't learn what we feel and know what it's like from a book, dietician, medical school, or from research findings.

I Didn't Get A Big Fat "Writing Bonus" From A Publisher, Nor Did I Have A "Ghost Writer"

<u>This</u> <u>book</u> <u>is</u> <u>the</u> <u>authentic,</u> <u>real</u> <u>story</u> <u>and</u> <u>discovery</u> of what I found and did to lose weight and reshape my body, as well as assist many people to do the same. I didn't get a monetary "bonus" from a publisher. <u>And</u> <u>unlike</u> <u>most</u> <u>of</u> <u>the</u> <u>other</u> <u>authors</u> <u>who</u> <u>have</u> <u>ghost</u> <u>writers</u> <u>help</u> <u>them</u> <u>write</u> <u>(or</u> <u>write</u> <u>the</u> <u>book</u> <u>for</u> <u>them),</u> *I <u>wrote</u> <u>every</u> <u>single</u> <u>word</u> <u>in</u> <u>this</u> <u>book</u> <u>myself.</u>* It may not be pretty, but it's real – and it works.

Also, you'll notice, I didn't pay or include a doctor to be a "co-author" for credibility or to make this book more "marketable" (this is what most publishers require an author like me to do). I refused to sell out and put *anyone* as a co-author who never experienced what you and I have, or who hasn't used this program.

<u>But</u> <u>please</u> <u>understand,</u> I do respect, reference, quote and speak about various medical professionals. I have many wonderful doctors, pharmacists and credentialed authorities as friends, co-workers, and associates; and without their assistance and support, my discovery and success would not have been possible.

...And I Chose Actual "Results" Over An Endorsement

Also, most publishers insist on having a forward from a credentialed person to add "credibility" to their book. Once again, I chose not to. Instead I chose to put <u>my</u> <u>results</u> and those of my clients in this book – and <u>let</u> <u>the</u> <u>actual</u> <u>results</u> <u>of</u> <u>previously</u> <u>over-</u><u>weight</u> <u>people</u> <u>like</u> <u>you</u> <u>speak</u> <u>for</u> <u>themselves.</u>

I Didn't Get Paid To Write This Book Nor Did I Do It To Sell Products

As you are about to learn in *The Discovery* section, this program was originally researched by me, and <u>only</u> <u>for</u> <u>my</u> <u>own</u> <u>per-</u><u>sonal</u> <u>use</u> for losing weight and improving the health challenges I had.

As people saw my results, they asked me to help them do

what I did. This led to the eventual writing of this book and my recommendation of a few products that I took alongside the eating and exercise programs I developed. Unlike other authors, I didn't get paid to write it, I was passionate about helping my friends and family lose weight and improve their health. Also, I didn't own a supplement company, nor did I have any plans to.

Years later, I eventually started a supplement company out of necessity, as I was concerned and wanted my readers to be assured they would be able to get the absolute best quality and effective products that were available. I cover all this in detail in the *Reference & Resource* section as it is a fascinating and inspiring story of how I went from being dead broke, and only having a dream and a passion to help others lose weight – to eventually being able to positively affect the health of over one million people worldwide!

The point of all this is that this book was originally written with only the pure intention of helping my friends, family, and all my new friends, like you, to lose weight and improve their health!

Now It's Just You and I...

This book is written probably unlike any weight loss book you have ever read. It's conversational, personal, moving, funny, sad, informative, and politically incorrect – and it's definitely not boring. *It's the real thing* – just straight forward information that works.

So pull up a chair, grab a cup of coffee, soda, or Twinkie (all of these your last!), and let's get acquainted – and let me assist you, like I have done with thousands of others, in losing weight and getting in the best shape of your life.

To Start Immediately

See the *Reshape Quick Start Guide* on the inside front cover...

The Discovery...

"How This Program Began
And Why It Will Work So Well For You"

Dear Friend,

I call you friend, because we both have probably had the same experiences and been on the same journey to lose weight (fat), keep it off, and improve our overall health.

Picture what you would look like if you were 5, 10, or even 20 or more pounds thinner. Imagine completely reshaping your body!

This happened to me - and it will happen for you also.

I have discovered the *real secret* to not only losing those ugly pounds - but keeping them off.

We've All Experienced This...

This powerful truth eluded me for some time. Maybe you have experienced what I have, and this will sound familiar to you.

For years, I struggled (and felt like I tortured myself at times) on many different diets. I spent thousands of dollars on many gimmicks and weight loss nutritional products. I bought books, answered ads and studied (which usually confused me more). All this time and money spent, with only mediocre results.

Sure, some of them worked OK. I'd work hard and only lose a few pounds after dieting for weeks and then... I'd go off it for just a weekend and BOOM - I would gain it all back (and sometimes even more) and feel bloated – and in only a couple of days. This just didn't seem fair, especially after sacrificing for all those weeks.

I began to resign myself to the belief that maybe I'd never get back to a decent, personally respectable shape.

A lot of my regular clothes just would not fit anymore. Sweat pants became my favorite clothes to wear since they expanded and were the only ones that did fit. I could have sworn someone came in my room when I wasn't there and moved some of the buttons closer. My belly just oozed over the sides of my pants, and I wasn't a happy camper – I had become a porkchop. The final straw was when I sat down on my couch one night, I saw my belly do this, "jiggle-back-and-forth" thing. Slightly amused (and mostly disgusted), I tapped my stomach with my hand and it sounded like a hollow watermelon!

Maybe all those people who said "once you're over 30 years old, your metabolism will never be the same - and you'll never be in shape like you used to be," were right. Feeling hopeless and discouraged – I started to believe them – until…

The Day That Changed My Life - And Body...

One day, I had an unanticipated meeting with a top sports doctor (who works with Olympic athletes), who was well versed on one of the hidden reasons why people don't lose weight on conventional diets (which I will cover shortly).

I combined some of her philosophies and recommendations with what I had just previously learned from two of the top weight loss and nutrition experts (and original pioneers) in the United States - and added the knowledge, concepts, and dieting techniques that I had learned throughout the years.

Fortunately everything I had done was not a complete waste of time or money, I just had to learn how to sort out what actually worked and eliminate what didn't work – and then incorporate it all together effectively – and almost overnight...

My body began to radically change – and...

Layers of Fat Started Peeling Off My Body!

Initially, some of the people close to me laughed at what I was doing. They said, "you can't eat something that good and lose weight." Some sarcastically questioned me, "How can you eat that much food and lose weight?" But I showed them - they were all wrong!

The results were so immediate and dramatic that other people (as well as myself) were shocked. I started burning fat so quickly that I can honestly remember at one point getting up in the morning and looking noticeably leaner from the previous day!

In less than 90 days I lost over 19 lbs. of ugly fat (that was the scale weight – I actually lost closer to 25 lbs), *over 4 inches from my waist*, and *another 9 inches* from the rest of my body, lowered my body fat and completely reshaped my body! I could see the results almost daily as my body began to change right before my eyes.

And best yet, I was able to keep the weight off and enjoy a normal life. I felt like I had the metabolism of a teenager. I was happy and comfortable with my body for the first time in years! *I had finally discovered the secret to not only losing weight, but keeping it off!* My energy levels were sky-high and I no longer felt sluggish and unmotivated.

Hey, What About Us?

Then something I never expected started to happen…

Seeing my dramatic results - my friends, family, and co-workers weren't laughing anymore - they were asking me if they could do what I had done. And guess what - it worked for them too! Friends and family, who like me had tried almost everything over the years, started losing weight and, more importantly, inches from all over their bodies! The best news is that I had never seen any other diet, weight loss plan or products work for some of these people. Based on actual results and real world experience, I can guarantee this will dramatically work for you too!

Because of these people, their results, and many other people who want similar results, you hold in your hands the finished work, which took tens of thousands of dollars and many years to discover.

What is contained in this book will work for you also!

What's My Method?

It's easy and makes perfect sense. **NO** zone this or high fat that. **NO** ridiculous lemonade, juice, or liquid diets. **NO** packaged meal plans or expensive clinics. **NO** harmful and unrealistic "do all, super-duper miracle" pills. **NO** high carbohydrate madness. **NO** all protein, no carbohydrate torture. **NO** food weighing. And best of all, **NO** complicated calorie counting!

The secret is actually a combination of scientifically proven principles that work - and one "essential element" that 99% of all other weight loss programs never mention or include. When I cover this in a moment, it will make perfect sense in understanding how your body works - and how you will lose weight immediately, safely and naturally.

One quick point - I'm not saying there aren't any other good diets or methods out there - there are. Almost all of them have a few good points, but I am unaware of any that have focused on this one upcoming "essential element" *and combined it with other key factors in the weight loss program I will share with you.* Based on results - if all these programs worked so well, the weight loss industry wouldn't have a 95% failure rate.

I know you are anxious to start. If you're like me, you are probably saying, "Just tell me what to eat, when to breathe and get outta my way!" Invest a few moments in reading the following pages so you understand what you are doing, how it works, and how to avoid the reasons why 95% of all diets fail.

Part of my goal is to educate you as well as give you the tools to reach your ideal weight. By learning these basic guidelines to eating – you may never have to diet again! This is not written as a medical publication and I'm not going to get technical with you. I'll keep it as basic as possible, using layman's terms - giving you just the facts (by the way, everything I'll tell you is scientifically and/or real world substantiated). So let's start with knowing...

What Types of Diets Don't Work...

If you are like me, at one time or another you've probably tried

My Reshape Results

"Your Clothes –
They Always Tell The Truth!"

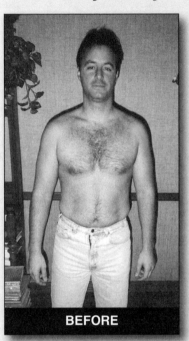

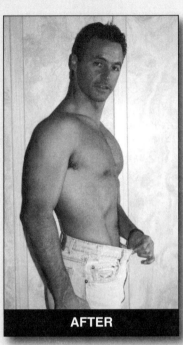

BEFORE

AFTER

No matter what the scale says, <u>your</u> <u>clothes</u> <u>are</u> <u>a</u> <u>more</u> <u>accurate</u> <u>gauge</u> <u>of</u> <u>your</u> <u>progress</u>.

Notice in the above photographs that <u>I</u> <u>am</u> <u>wearing</u> <u>the</u> <u>same</u> <u>jeans</u>. In the before picture, my stomach is "oozing over," and in the after picture, my pants are loose with inches to spare! Although you can't see it, the hips and legs are much looser also. This is one way to tell you are *losing fat*, and not water and muscle.

Although I lost over 19 pounds, my skin and muscles are tighter, toned, and more defined. This is the look of healthy weight loss (losing fat, not muscle). On this program you will lose <u>only</u> <u>fat</u>, and will have this toned, reshaped look. In the after picture, notice how much healthier my eyes and face look! In the before picture, I wasn't a happy camper – I really did feel as bad as my face looks.

one, two, or all of these. I think at one point, I probably used them all together to try to get results!

These are the types of diets that don't work:

- Extremely low calorie diets
- Rapid weight loss plans
- Liquid diets (except if medically administered)
- Starvation diets
- Appetite suppressants
- Complicated diets where you need to know food portions, sizes, types - and need a scale, a compass and a road map to keep track of everything
- Lemonade, juice, or single food diets
- **Diets that don't correct the digestive system and restore the intestinal tract**
- **Diets where the preservation and support of muscle is not emphasized**
- **Carbohydrate dominant diets**

And, I want to emphasize one very important point regarding weight loss: In the past we have heard many weight loss professionals and governmental agencies promote carbohydrate dominant diets (I'll define and explain this in the next section), stating that dietary fat is the problem. Well here's the fact:

> "Americans reduced their fat intake during the past decade by 25%, yet in this same time, the number of overweight people *increased by 33%!*"

A fact even more sad is that, "since 1980, the percentage of children (1-12) and young adults (12-19) who are overweight has doubled!" If this trend of carbohydrate dominant diets worked so well, then three out of four (75%) Americans would not be overweight.

The truth is that high carbohydrate diets will make you fat!

They can also cause many other health problems, such as high cholesterol, diabetes, cardiovascular problems, and other degenerative diseases.

What you are about to see is not a high fat - no carbohydrate diet, but a program that restores the body to optimum health, so you can enjoy carbohydrate foods. It will also educate you so you can enjoy foods that we have all been taught to avoid!

Seven Reasons Why These and Most Diets Don't Work...

The reason these and other diets fail is:

1. They focus on losing weight instead of body fat (I made a point of previously telling you I lost body fat, over 13 inches, and 19 scale pounds vs. 25 total pounds for a reason).

2. They cause you to lose muscle along with fat (remember this as we cover the Yo-Yo syndrome).

3. They do nothing to correct one of the main reasons why people have trouble losing or fail to lose weight - which is their digestive system and colon related problems!

4. They do not cleanse your system; but usually cause a build up of "matter" (also called mucoid plaque) in the intestinal tract - which attributes to bloating (covered shortly).

5. They do not treat other underlying problems that can be the real cause of being overweight, like Candida albicans (covered shortly), or insulin resistance (covered in the next section).

6. They do not discover and remedy common food intolerances and allergies that cause bloating and prevent weight loss (covered in next section).

7. They do not address or correct hormone imbalances or declines (covered in the next section).

Also, *low calorie diets (which this is not) usually reduce a person's metabolism by 15-30%.* This is why you will normally feel tired, listless, and run down. The most common cause of this is a loss of vital and healthy muscle (which we will cover in a moment). When you maintain - and especially develop more muscle - your metabolism increases - and you burn more fat!

Diets that don't work cause you to:

1. Lose water weight (one reason for rapid weight loss).

2. Lose muscle (which you should not lose).

3. Slow down your metabolism (i.e. low calorie).

4. Impair your metabolism (appetite suppressants and especially stimulants - such as *Ma Huang, Ephedra, Caffeine, White Willow Bark, Kola Nut, Guarana, Etc...*)

Note: Consumers typically report that they suffer sluggish metabolisms and gain weight after using stimulants.

Most of the diets previously mentioned can be worse than not dieting at all - because you end up with more body fat and an impaired digestive system!

Why Muscle Is The SECRET To Healthy, Long-Term Weight Loss - And A Firm, Toned Body...

I once read how one health professional estimated that: *1 out of every 3-4 pounds lost on a diet is muscle!*

Most people do not realize how dangerous this is since your heart and organs are muscle (also known as "lean body mass" or "lean body tissue"). Your digestive tract (key point in a few moments), cardiac action, and pulsing of your arteries all involve smooth muscle activity.

Your heart being the leanest muscle of all!

Do you really want to lose muscle (lean body tissue) on a diet? NO, NO, NO - but this is one common problem with most diets and the reason people experience the "Yo-Yo Syndrome," which is the gaining back of the weight you lost (with usually more fat).

How To Naturally Increase Your Metabolism And Turn Your Body Into A Fat-Burning Machine...

Always remember this: *Muscle increases your metabolism! Muscle loss slows down your metabolism.*

Muscle burns calories. It can help turn your body into a "fat-burning furnace!" This is why you do not want to lose muscle, but instead to gain muscle on a good diet (remember this when I give you advice on weighing yourself and what to do with your scale).

Muscle tissue loss in our bodies is also part of the aging process. Muscle retention and the addition of muscle (especially in women) can combat aging, and also create a firm, toned body, like when you were younger.

This is one reason why my clients who use this system have youthful and healthy looking bodies compared to how other people look after using those popular, faddish weight loss programs and supplements.

There are two ways to maintain and/or gain muscle:

1. By exercising, preferably with some type of resistance exercise (some diets hit this one right on but miss this next one), and

2. By making sure your body gets a good supply of usable amino acids/protein (to ensure a positive nitrogen balance), so you can maintain and build muscle tissue.

Four ways to achieve this second one are: 1) through a new medically used and scientifically proven product I found which we will discuss called *AminoSculpt*; 2) by structuring your dieting and eating certain muscle supporting foods (this is what I do in the *Eating Plan Section*); 3) by helping your body to naturally optimize its Growth Hormone levels (covered in the next section); and 4) by including a quality and cost-efficient protein meal-replacement drink. I'm not saying you should not exercise - I have a whole section on covering this - but realistically, I know some people don't and/or won't exercise.

While using this system and losing fat, I have personally worked with and witnessed people who used *AminoSculpt* and did not exercise - who ended up gaining muscle! Now don't worry (especially if you are a woman) - if you gain muscle, you're not going to look like a big bulky bodybuilder - your body will reshape, and will look and be firmer and toned like when you were younger!

Personally, on this program, when I lost 19 pounds – none of it was muscle (see my photos). This is highly unusual on most diets.

The "Most Important Fat Loss & Body Shaping Element" That Guarantees Results
And That 99% Of All Other Programs Overlook...

The following *"essential body-shaping element"* is one of the most successful concepts I have learned in general health and weight loss. It took over 6 years to discover the best, long term way to utilize this essential body shaping element. *Ninety-nine percent of all weight loss programs and most health professionals miss this one topic completely!* Finally, after years of research and trial and error, I mastered this with the right combination of foods and nutritional aids.

> *"The powerful truth and answer to most of your weight loss challenges and general health problems lies in the center of your body - **in your colon and intestinal tract.**"*

What you are about to learn is a healthy way to lose between 4-20 pounds on top of the fat loss you will experience! Plus, you can reduce or eliminate bloating and your waist can flatten or reduce by an inch or two! With most individuals this can be almost immediate! After you correct this - the fat can melt off even more rapidly.

Let me start to explain this to you by the use of a unique story:

One day all the body parts got together to discuss <u>who</u> <u>is</u> <u>the</u> <u>most</u> <u>important</u> - and who would be the head spokesperson for the body. The first to speak was the eyes. The eyes said, "We're the most important. Without us, the rest of the body couldn't see where it is going or get around!" The ears then spoke up and said, "We think we're the most important, we enable the body to hear what is happening in the world!" The arms and legs said, "No, we are the most important. We protect the body and groom it with our hands. We enable the body to move around!" The mouth spoke up and said, "I'm the most important, I feed the body and communicate with others." Then the brain spoke up and said, "No, you've all forgotten how important I am. I think and make all the decisions for the whole body. I decide important things!" The skin spoke, "You've all forgotten. I am the largest organ in the body - I protect it. I am the most important."

The last to speak was the anus, who also represented his <u>adjoining</u> <u>part</u> and friend, the colon. The anus timidly said, "I think I should be considered for the most important." All the other body parts laughed at the anus and said, "You are definitely not the most important, why should we even consider you?" Hurt and rejected, the anus left the discussion and thought, "I'll show them." The anus, then shut himself off and refused to work. The other body parts thought nothing of it and went on their way. Nothing happened at first, but after a few days, the other body parts didn't quite feel the same as before - **they felt worse**.

And after a few more days, strange things began to happen:

The eyes became blurry and tired - and started to lose their vision. The ears started ringing, and began to lose their hearing. The arms and legs became sluggish and tired - and felt too heavy to move. Their joints became achy and very painful - and mobility was lost. The mouth became parched and developed a coating. The brain became confused and foggy. And the skin lost its youthful and healthy shine - developing "breakouts" of pimples, acne and rashes. The skin also began to push out and expand as fat began to accumulate all over.

All the toxic build-up that was normally excreted began to overflow throughout the body - <u>rapidly</u> <u>aging</u> <u>and</u> <u>slowly</u> <u>killing</u> <u>it</u>.

It was a hard lesson, but it was only then that the other body parts discovered <u>who</u> <u>was</u> <u>the</u> <u>most</u> <u>important</u> <u>and</u> <u>critical</u> <u>to</u> <u>their</u> <u>overall</u> <u>health</u> <u>and</u> <u>in</u> <u>maintaining</u> <u>the</u> <u>body's</u> <u>young</u>, <u>beautiful</u> <u>shape</u> <u>and</u> <u>appearance</u>.

This story is a more graphic way of showing <u>how important the colon and digestive system is to your overall health and weight loss</u>. The body's inability to digest and absorb vital nutrients, and eliminate waste products and toxins can severely affect your health and weight loss.

Now let's take a look at how this can affect and accelerate weight loss.

Can You Really Lose 4-20 Pounds Without Dieting?

I'll walk you through this and keep it as simple as possible:

When you eat foods, drink water and breathe air, you are exposed to and ingest various toxins, chemicals and pollutants. <u>You cannot avoid them - they are everywhere</u>. These items cannot always be eliminated and can lodge in your intestinal tract and cells of your body (fat cells are great holding tanks of toxins). On top of all that, there are certain foods like white flours (breads, pastas, etc.) which have <u>processed</u> ingredients your body <u>cannot</u> digest. Some preservatives in food do not break down either. Mucus forming foods like dairy products (milk) can also complicate matters. And over-eating, alcohol, and sugars can contribute as well.

Even if you were to eat perfectly, auto and other pollution in the air you breathe can build up in your system. Water sources, even filtered ones, can also contain many contaminants.

Over time, all these toxins, chemicals, preservatives, pollutants, processed foods, and indigestible ingredients – build up in the intestinal tract and in the cells of your body. This build-up (also referred to as "mucoid plaque") also consists of excess mucus and old, uneliminated fecal matter. Some foods you are eating don't completely digest and can putrefy in the intestinal tract causing problems - as these waste matters and toxins re-circulate throughout the body.

Because of this build-up, problems like improper elimination and constipation occur. This build-up even prevents your body from absorbing the crucial nutrients in food that give life to your body!

Reshape Success Story: Kirsten

"She Lost Over 5½ Inches In Only 27 Days!"

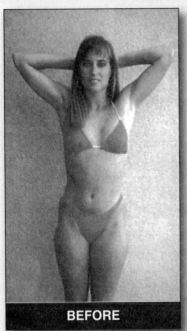

BEFORE

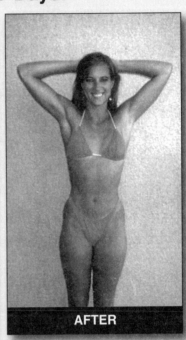

AFTER

When I first learned about cleansing, I coached my friend, Kirsten, on a similar, less developed program. The cleansing product used was about one-half as effective as the cleansing product, *Sculpt n' Cleanse*, I now recommend.

Kirsten had never cleansed, or done any exercise or dieting for four years prior. In only 27 days, she lost about 2 ½ inches from her waist, almost 3 inches from her hips and thighs, inches from all over the rest of her body and completely reshaped her physique. You can even see a noticeable difference in her face!

Kirsten followed a *Plan B* eating program (which was before I refined the *Eating Plan A*, which accelerates weight loss), and substituted 1-2 protein shakes per day in place of meals. For exercise Kirsten used weights 2-3 times per week (for the first time in her life), and did some light aerobic work on a trampoline rebounder for the other 2-3 days.

Even if you eliminate regularly, this build-up is still taking place.

The average person can have between 4-20 pounds of this toxic matter built up in their system (Note: some health experts report that the build-up can be between 7-25 pounds, but I've chosen to be more conservative).

On top of this, poisons, germs, parasites and worms can accumulate on the walls of the colon. As a result of all this, toxin poisoning can be absorbed into the bloodstream and circulate throughout the body. Also, the development of unfriendly bacteria like Candida albicans can develop (covered next).

The poisons from the "build-up" can *weaken and stress the heart; can cause skin problems like blemishes, pimples, psoriasis, wrinkling and other skin conditions; can cause bad breath; can cause weakness, cramping, and fatigue in the muscles; can cause stiffness and pain in the joints; can cause brain and mental problems; and can be responsible for many allergies, sinus and other related conditions.*

Degenerative conditions of the kidneys, colon, as well as indigestion, headaches, irritability, dizziness, depression, fatigue, arthritis, menstrual problems, and insomnia may result from these accumulations of toxins in the body.

Ok, Ok, So What Do I Do
to Get This "TOXIC STUFF" Out?

The only effective way I have found to get this build-up out of your system is to do a "cleansing program".

A *cleansing program* usually consists of: 1) a cleansing supplement, 2) following a specific eating plan for a limited amount of time, and 3) drinking plenty of pure water.

The best supplement on the market I have used for cleansing is *Sculpt n' Cleanse*. This product is time-tested with close to one million satisfied users and will quickly and effectively rid your body of the built-up matter lodged in the intestinal tract. Many of my clients also notice it helps to alleviate bloating, and they lose weight and flatten their waistline quicker.

While cleansing, you eliminate more frequently for a period of time as the waste matter is broken down and removed from your system. But unlike other cleansing supplements available, *Sculpt n' Cleanse* is gentle and will not interfere with your daily schedule.

Some people will find they lose anywhere from a couple of pounds and up to ten or more (based on how much build-up you have and how overweight you are)! Typically, the more overweight a person is, the greater amount of built-up matter is in their system.

Your Waistline Will Just Flatten!

Another fantastic benefit is as this build-up is removed from your system, you will probably find that your waistline or abdominal area literally "flattens," or is reduced by as much as a few inches!

A lot of time, feeling bloated or having a tummy that protrudes is <u>not</u> only from fat on the outside, <u>but</u> <u>largely</u> <u>from</u> <u>the</u> <u>built</u>-<u>up</u> <u>matter</u> <u>pushing</u> <u>outward</u> <u>from</u> <u>the</u> <u>inside</u>!

A Quick Test

Grab your tummy with your hands. If you do not grab much fat, but your stomach bulges out like you swallowed a melon (or when you tap your hands on your tummy and it sounds like a hollow melon - like mine did), or it protrudes and/or is not completely flat; then you probably have this intestinal build-up or something causing bloating, and/or some type of intestinal problem, like Candida.

If you grab handfuls of fat (sounds pleasant, huh?) and still, your abdominal muscles are flat - then you are mainly fat (although you still have toxins and some build-up, and will notice a significant difference from cleansing).

When I was in school, I used to wrestle. Although I would get my body fat low and my stomach muscles would show - my stomach would still "round-out" or protrude. I wasn't fat, but my waistline would not flatten no matter how much I dieted or exercised that area.

When I learned about cleansing and did it - **for the first time since my youth, my stomach came in and went completely flat!** The reason was that I had just eliminated the built-up intestinal matter. Many people I have counseled have also experienced tremendous and immediate results from this.

Regular Diets Don't Even Come Close to Explaining or Doing This...

A really important point is that this type of cleansing is only possible with an herbal cleansing product, such as *Sculpt n' Cleanse*.

Some other diets will claim, "our diet has sufficient fiber in the foods for that purpose." Fiber in foods and fiber supplements are helpful and I recommend them, but alone they cannot break down the build-up like an herbal cleansing supplement. Fiber does play a role in cleansing by helping the absorption and elimination of toxins, but the ultimate breakdown and removal will only come from a quality cleansing supplement like *Sculpt n' Cleanse*.

Fiber is essential for weight loss and general health. That is why I recommend a new medically used, fiber supplement called *Ready Fiber* (the world's first liquid fiber), especially *since most people are fiber deficient* – with 9 out of 10 Americans not getting the daily recommended amount of fiber. *Ready Fiber's* super-concentrated formula (12 grams per single ounce vs. 3 grams per eight ounces of the leading fiber brands) will ensure you get enough to affect weight loss. Unlike most other fiber products *Ready Fiber* also contains *prebiotics*, which help stimulate the growth of beneficial "good" bacteria in the colon, which is important when cleansing and fighting Candida.

Most cleansing products on the market are too harsh on the body or do not work well (see my discussion of this in the *Supplement Section*). I recommend only tried and true products, like *Sculpt n'*

Cleanse, that are proven to work, strengthen the body's own natural processes, and also can help the process of ridding the body of unfriendly bacteria like Candida albicans.

The Other Overlooked Weight Loss Enemy - Candida albicans...

A large part of the population has Candida albicans (Candida) and is unaware of it. If you have been trying to lose weight unsuccessfully - or have other nagging health problems - there is a good chance <u>Candida</u> - <u>along</u> <u>with</u> <u>many</u> <u>other</u> <u>problems</u> <u>it</u> <u>may</u> <u>be</u> <u>causing</u> <u>you</u> - <u>is</u> <u>why</u>.

Very few diets ever mention this either - and if you have it – and do not take specific actions - it really will not matter how good your diet is, or how much you exercise.

What is Candida albicans?

There are 80 species, but the one most commonly discussed in medical literature is Candida albicans (we will refer to it as "*Candida*"). Simply put, Candida is a mold and yeast fungus that naturally resides primarily in the colon, but can also live in the mouth, throat, and vagina. Candida and other *unfriendly* bacteria are balanced by *friendly* "lactobacteria".

A few important facts to know about Candida are that:

1. It can increase beyond normal levels and cause *weight gain*, bloating, as well as digestive and other problems,

2. It is unable to produce its own food, so it depends on what you eat, and

3. *It feeds on sugars - which basically means* <u>*carbohydrates*</u>.

What Causes Candida albicans?

Much of Candida overgrowth is caused by the use of

antibiotic drugs (for any reason - illness or even as a treatment for acne when younger), **birth control pills or steroids, poor diet (especially those containing a lot of sugars - carbohydrates), nutrient deficiencies, increased toxic exposure, and stress.**

How It Can Affect You...

This book is concerned with fat loss and body shaping - and one of the major causes that prevents this is Candida!

Weight gain, problems losing weight and/or keeping it off are very common, but look at what else is related to Candida:

Indigestion, constipation, bloating, diarrhea, abdominal discomfort, gastritis, mucus in the stool, itchy or scaly skin, acne, rashes, distorted vision, tearing or inflamed eyes, pain or fluid in the ears, deafness, reoccurring ear infections, sore or bleeding gums, dry mouth, recurring bladder infections, burning or urgent urination, fatigue, loss of hair, insomnia, loss of appetite, irritability, mood swings, head-aches, memory or brain related problems, allergies, sinus congestion, painful joints, vaginal yeast overgrowth, sugar or alcohol cravings.

Most people are treating symptoms they have (like the above) directly, **not the underlying cause**, which can be (and in a lot of cases is) Candida.

You may have Candida or yeast overgrowth if you also *"feel sick all over;" have colds and flus that keep coming back; experience continual fatigue, general malaise and loss of energy or libido; get frequent vaginal or yeast infections or bladder infections; are bothered by food sensitivities; crave sugar (or alcohol-which is primarily carbohydrates or sugars); experience depression or irritability; have frequent headaches; suffer from digestive problems such as bloating, gas, intestinal cramps, or indigestion; are sensitive to tobacco smoke, perfume, and other chemicals; and have a protruding lower tummy!*

(Source: Some of the preceding information on Candida was based on information from "Natural Healing" by Joan A. Freidrich, Ph.D., C.C.N.).

Oh No, Some of This Sounds Like Me - What Do I Do?

Like with any serious health problem, you should always consult a qualified health professional who is versed on treating Candida.

The purpose of mentioning this is to make you <u>aware</u> <u>of</u> <u>a</u> <u>common</u> <u>underlying</u> <u>problem</u> <u>that</u> <u>may</u> <u>hamper</u> <u>your</u> <u>weight</u> <u>loss</u>. In my experience, this was never brought up to me until my friend, Dr. Vicky Vodon, educated me about it.

The *Eating Plans* coming up in this book are formulated - *not only for proper weight loss, but for combating Candida* - if it is present. By following these plans, you will get a double effect like I did. <u>This</u> <u>is</u> <u>one</u> <u>of</u> <u>the</u> <u>reasons</u> <u>why</u> <u>certain</u> <u>foods</u> <u>are</u> <u>limited</u> <u>or</u> <u>avoided</u> <u>at</u> <u>first</u>.

Due to an overexposure to highly processed foods, especially carbohydrates (chips, breads, cereals, white flour products, pizzas, pastas, candy, sodas, etc.) and sugars, people have developed Candida and damaged their sugar metabolism which enables them to properly process and digest these foods when eaten. The good news is that you do not have to give these foods up forever - although you should be aware of and at least try to limit them after your system is restored and your weight is lost.

Remember, <u>Candida</u> <u>is</u> <u>a</u> <u>live</u> <u>microorganism</u> <u>within</u> <u>you</u> <u>that</u> <u>feeds</u> <u>off</u> <u>of</u> <u>sugars</u> – which is what *carbohydrates* are broken down into! This is <u>one</u> <u>reason</u> why some types of carbohydrates are restricted in the eating plans, and then gradually introduced back into your diet.

For <u>Ultimate</u> and <u>Assured</u> Results...

Controlled eating is not the only way to combat Candida and digestive related problems. Cleansing with an effective product like *Sculpt n' Cleanse* will also assist this. *Sculpt n' Cleanse* is a powerful supplement and should <u>always</u> <u>be</u> <u>"the</u> <u>first</u> <u>step"</u> <u>when</u> <u>starting</u> <u>any</u> <u>weight</u> <u>loss</u> <u>program</u>.

MSM and *Ready Fiber* are other supplements that can be added to help combat Candida and digestive related problems (see the *Supplement Section*).

Cleansing <u>Plus</u> an Eating Plan Equals...

As mentioned earlier, if you combine cleansing with a specific *Eating Plan* (like shown in *Plan A or B*), the results will astound you.

The upcoming recommended *Eating Plans* are effective and are designed a little differently than regular cleansing programs. These recommended eating plans not only support cleansing, but are designed for weight loss, to re-establish a healthy carbohydrate sugar metabolism, to help rid your body of unfriendly bacteria like Candida albicans, to combat common food intolerances and allergies, to balance and improve hormone levels, and to help restore your digestive process.

Combine all these with a little exercise - and get ready for the magic show! <u>You are going to transform and reshape your body quicker than, and like never before!</u> What all this means is that you will finally be able to lose weight and keep it off because you are also correcting some underlying problems – beyond dieting – that prevent many people from losing weight.

You'll Get Results Too!

What all this adds up to is RESULTS! Just to summarize, here is what to expect:

- Lose body <u>fat</u> (not muscle)

- Firm and tone your body by maintaining your muscle (or even gaining some)

- Increase your metabolism (and restore it to more youthful levels)

- Increase your energy levels

- Improve digestion - and get relief from common digestive

Reshape Success Story: Dawn

"48 Year-Old Woman Now Has A Body Better Than Most Women In Their 20's"

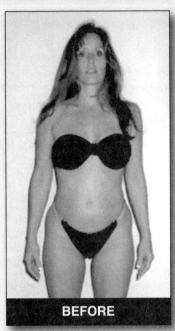

BEFORE

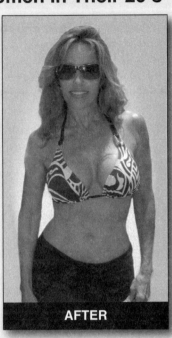

AFTER

For years, Dawn had been able to stay in shape, but she eventually gained, what she called, that extra "hard-to-lose" weight in her 40's. Dawn used this program including, *Sculpt n' Cleanse, AminoSculpt,* and *Ready Fiber.* In Dawn's words, here's what she experienced:

"Sculpt n' Cleanse helped my bloating and waistline trim down quickly. Now, I still use it any time I need to flatten my waistline, and when I eat heavier meals, or go on vacation – it works fast! AminoSculpt helped me lose weight, and tone my body. I even sleep better with it and my skin is softer and smoother."

"Also, I've had digestive problems since I was a young girl. Many foods make me nauseous, bloated, give me a greasy feeling, and make my stomach spasm. The first time I used Ready Fiber, my stomach spasms and greasy feeling immediately went away! Now I use Ready Fiber regularly, and it calms my stomach, and I don't get the bloating or cramping."

For exercise, Dawn did power (fast-paced) walking, and some light dumbbell exercises at home. You can see a difference in Dawn's face, chest, arms, legs; and her waistline is flat and hip bulges are gone.

Note: Also see Dawn's photos on the cover and in the Exercise Descriptions

The Discovery...

How to Completely Reshape Your Body   27

problems like bloating and occasional constipation

- Better absorption of foods and supplements

- Increase your overall health

- Better awareness of which foods are good for you and those you should avoid

- *You will RESHAPE your body, look and feel younger, and will appear more attractive*

The Four Simple Steps
That Guarantee Your Success...

One reason this program will work for you is that it contains a *multi-disciplinarian approach.*

This means a comprehensive approach for attacking fat from many different angles - and starting with the most important – your colon.

The *Four Simple Steps* that are synergistically combined to melt off ugly fat are:

1. An exact, deliberate *eating program* (rather than a "diet"),

2. Specific and highly effective *supplementation,*

3. *Exercise,* and

4. Nutritional *education and knowledge* (the information in this book and my website: **www.reshapeforlife.com**).

Important Point

This program is designed to be flexible. The *Four Simple Steps* are basic principles that everyone should do, so I recommend them all for quick and highly effective results. Realistically, I know some people will not or do not want to do some, so this program is also designed so you can still get the results you want even if you do some things differently. This will be discussed in detail throughout the book.

If you decide to use all or most of these steps, get ready to change and completely reshape your body. If you use some of them, you can still achieve your goals – just understand that it might take a little longer.

A Key Point About Inclusion of Recommended Supplements in This Program

I have seen and heard a few weight loss programs on the market that say, "All you need to do is follow this diet and you'll get all the nutrients you'll need" or "no popping any pills or potions here," or "our program accomplishes 'that' by the foods we've included." I'll be very blunt: these are ludicrous statements containing uninformed nutritional and weight loss philosophies.

In the *Eating Plan and Supplement Sections*, I will present some very compelling facts on why you should supplement.

Furthermore, why wouldn't you want to take perfectly safe, all-natural supplements that have been clinically and medically substantiated (some with U.S. patents) to work? Especially nowadays, when it is highly unlikely we get enough of the critical nutrients we need from the foods we eat.

As for me personally, when it comes to weight loss – if I was in Los Angeles, I'd rather drive a car (use supplements) to Las Vegas than walk there (not use them). Good, proven supplements make the trip faster and more enjoyable. We'll cover this thoroughly in the *Supplement Section*.

One Last Thing to Consider: *"90 vs. 3,650"*

Consider for a moment everything you have put in your body for the last 10 years (that's approximately 3,650 days). Some of you might even want to look back even further.

Picture the foods you've eaten. Look back at the holidays when we all overdo it a little (but isn't that second serving on Thanksgiving so good – until afterwards). Remember some of the birthdays or special events, vacations and parties you attended. We all have eaten the same things at one time or another – we're only human – apple pie, chocolate (ever notice how you start with one Hershey's Kiss or M&M and end up eating the whole bag?), pizza, sodas, diet sodas, breads, chips, crackers, those orange cheeses that are not naturally orange, pasteurized milk, dips, cakes, beer, wine, deli and lunch meats, cereals (remember downing a couple of bowls at a time as a kid), meats, chicken, canned foods – the list can go on forever. And has anyone breathed any air or drank any water (that wasn't distilled) lately?

Feeling guilty? Don't, you are just human like the rest of the population – and it's the way a lot of us were raised. What matters is *what you do now* with this new knowledge that can transform your body and improve your health. And best yet...

Now, here is the comforting part and a key question:

That's it – *90 days*! You can see tremendous results in 90 days!

Isn't it comforting to know that after all you have done in the last 3,650 days, you can completely alter your body in such a short period of time – and for the rest of your life?

> **"Whether you have dieted at all before or not, can you commit to only 90 DAYS to help correct what has happened to your body over the last 3,650 days?"**

For some of you who are not too far out of shape or for those who just want to tune up – you'll probably get there in a lot less time – 2 weeks, 30 or 60 days – although I encourage you to complete a 90 day cycle to help restore your body.

For others, who are just "not in too good of shape" – it's ok, we can say it among friends – you just plain let yourself go and gave up (because no one ever showed or explained to you an effective way to lose weight). With this program you'll see great results in 90 days – and it is just going to take a little longer to get all the results you want. Realistically, you can only physically lose so much weight in a healthy way over a given period of time. But, by doing another 90 day cycle, you'll continue to get great results – and they will come much quicker and easier!

For me, I achieved much more than I set out to do in just 90 days. Initially, I was looking to drop a few pounds – but ended up shedding 19 unwanted pounds of fat and lost 13 inches from all over my body, while adding muscle and reshaping my physique – all at the same time. I no longer get bloated when I eat certain foods, my bowel movements are regular, my milk (lactose) allergies have subsided, little nagging aches and pains went away, and my energy levels shot through the roof! All it took was 90 days – and I didn't try to take any short-cuts (although I will show you how I "cheated" along the way)!

Not to mention, no one gave me a book or program like this – you get a head start!

By the way, it really didn't take me 90 days to achieve my results – I lost almost all of the weight and inches in a little over 60 days! I stayed on this program for 90 days strict – like I encourage you to – to fine tune my body, and more importantly, to restore my digestive system. This will help to prevent gaining weight back and really increase your metabolism.

Oh My, Nothing's Happening!

OK, some of you are probably a little impatient like me. Whenever I've dieted, and even when I started this program – I looked into the mirror after about 5-7 days (and for me that's being patient; it's usually 3 days) – and thought, "Oh my, NOTHING'S HAPPENING!"

Then I actually thought about it. It took me longer than 7 days or even 90 days to get out of shape – **so why should I honestly expect it to go away overnight?** Keep this in mind: *"Lose it overnight – gain it back overnight. Lose it right – keep it off for good."*

Well, let me share something exciting with you. When you restore your body from the inside out, you hit a momentum period where your body will amaze you at how quickly it changes. Your health is like compounding interest (and it can go either way). It may not look like your body's changing much at first, but then the results quadruple! I can remember mornings where I woke up – and looked and felt thinner and more firm and shapely from only the night before! For some of you it will be quicker. For me it took about 6 weeks (halfway). So take it one step at a time.

The reason I tell you my story and will share pieces of it throughout this book is because I, like you, have done the same things and have struggled with the same issues. Since I originally used and developed this program, it has worked for many other people – **and it will work for you too!**

This book contains what I did, what I used, how I did it, and some fine-tuning and improvements I have continued to learn over the years to help my clients achieve even better results.

You now have a clear picture of what you need to do to lose fat, reshape you body, and restore your health. In your hands you hold the knowledge and the road map that shows you how to do this.

So all you have left to do is **start** and follow what is laid out for you.

I know you will do well... SO START!

Best wishes and may God's blessings be with you along the way.

Jim Caras

Jim Caras, Author

Eating Plans

Always consult a physician
before starting any diet or
nutritional program.

"Eating Right To Reshape Your Body For Life!"

This section is about most people's favorite subject and past time: *food and eating.*

Knowing that your goal is to lose weight (fat), reshape your body, and achieve optimum health and energy, let's start with a simple and universal principle that <u>will</u> <u>determine</u> <u>your</u> <u>health</u> <u>and</u> <u>weight</u> <u>control</u> <u>for</u> <u>the</u> **<u>rest</u>** **<u>of</u>** **<u>your</u>** **<u>life</u>**:

> *"What **YOU** put into your body will determine how <u>you</u> <u>look</u> and <u>feel</u>, and your <u>overall</u> <u>health</u>."*

The bottom line is nutrition – the food you eat and its <u>quality</u> is the key determining factor of your health. Once again, it is an <u>investment</u> you make in yourself.

This simple concept, if mastered, will bring you great joy, happiness, and the body you have always wanted.

Your first step in mastering and developing your new body is to know that there are:

<u>NO</u> Diets Here!

This program involves an *"eating"* program, <u>not</u> a diet!

The difference can be found in the first three letters of each word above: DIE vs. EAT

DIE (in <u>D</u> <u>I</u> <u>E</u> T) describes most programs really well, since that is what you feel is happening when you are cutting calories and torturing yourself.

With this program, you are just going to be EATING – the right foods and enough of them to change your metabolism, reshape your body, and improve your health.

Wait – Don't Eat Yet...

I know you're anxious to get started. Before you start swinging your forks and spoons, let's take a quick moment for me to explain two critical areas that will make this process easier for you…

…AVOID The Foods That "Explode" In Your Stomach, Wreak Havoc In Your Body, And Pack On Fat!

The two upcoming sections, *"Nine Ways These Eating Plans Help You Shed Fat and Avoid Nagging Health Problems"* and *"Food 101,"* will teach you the why, what and when of eating smart. Most people who have dieted, read weight loss books, gone to expensive clinics, or used exotic supplements really don't know this information, so you'll be a big step ahead in losing weight.

This information will also help you navigate through the mess and confusion of choosing effective and safe weight loss and nutritional supplements, as you will now understand what types can safely and effectively work with your body's own natural processes.

Many authors make this type of information sooooo long and confusing. I know you're just trying to lose some weight, and not put a man on the moon, so I'll avoid the scientific dissertation - and at the risk of offending the dieticians and academics - I'll keep it as basic, simple, and fun as I can.

If you have ever had trouble losing weight and keeping it off – the following will explain why…

The upcoming eating plans are designed to restore the body and address the common problems - *unknown to most people* - that prevent them from successfully losing weight and keeping it off.

By taking a few moments to review the following information you will learn how to:

1. Use food as a weight loss and health improvement *tool*, and
2. Limit or avoid foods that cause your body problems.

You'll Be Attacking Fat And Restoring Your Body 9 Different Ways...

Here is why these eating programs work so well and how they do it. While some of these topics were covered in the first section of this book, I will expand more on the ones that were not.

These eating plans optimize your health and weight loss by helping you:

1. **CLEANSE** and remove the built up matter (mucoid plaque) and toxins from your body. As covered previously, this is done when using a cleansing oriented eating program combined with a cleansing supplement, like *Sculpt n' Cleanse*.

2. **BUILD** and preserve muscle for a firmer, toned and more youthful looking body. Remember, muscle weighs 22% more than fat, so you can lose those excess pounds and reshape your body into a beautiful new you – even though your scale weight hasn't changed much. Don't worry, you are losing fat. Use a tape measure and how you look to determine your progress and results, *not a scale*.

3. **BURN** fat and increase your metabolism. More muscle also means a higher metabolism and that you'll be able to eat more food! Combine that with a new body that is not bogged down

Eating Plans

with toxins, and you'll feel great and have more energy. The foods you will be eating will help your body burn fat (more of this in the next few points).

The upcoming *Eating Plans* also address the following bodily functions and problem areas that sabotage most people's weight loss:

4. Candida:

Candida and its negative effects on weight loss and the body were covered in the first section. *Eating Plan A* is also a basic eating regimen to help correct the overgrowth of yeast and bacteria.

5. Food Sensitivities:

Many people unknowingly have food intolerances or allergies. For these people, certain common foods can cause adverse reactions in the body. Over 100 health conditions can be caused or worsened by food sensitivities. Reactions to these foods can occur within hours to days after being eaten, making this weight loss and health roadblock difficult to identify.

Most people notice the adverse effects of these foods in three areas: 1) *gastrointestinal* (bloating, constipation, gas, and irritable bowel conditions); 2) *neurological* (migraines and headaches), and 3) *dermatological* (eczema, psoriasis, and other skin conditions). Continuous consumption of these foods weakens your immune system, causing a myriad of other health problems. And for the main purpose of this book, they can prevent weight loss.

A very common food intolerance is with glutens, which are contained in certain grains (carbohydrates) like wheat, rye, and barley. These and other foods have been avoided in the upcoming *Eating Plans*.

Other common foods that people have intolerances with are: milk or dairy, sugar, peanuts, soy, eggs, corn, glycerin (in protein bars), and artificial sweeteners, especially aspartame. In the *Eating Plans*, some of these are avoided and the less common ones are included (eggs), or are limited (corn). I have found that most people can tolerate these, so I have included them, but if you know you have an intolerance with a specific food, then eliminate it. If you notice any of the previously mentioned effects after a few weeks on this or any diet, then eliminate a commonly eaten food group (like all dairy), for a week or two and see if the condition clears. If so, you'll know to avoid that food or food group. Also try organic and/or raw foods that are not altered (i.e. without pesticides, added hormones, antibiotics, irradiation, homogenization, etc.). *Sometimes it's not the foods that are causing you problems, but how they are processed and treated prior to consumption.*

6. **Insulin Resistance:**

If <u>you</u> <u>have</u> <u>had</u> <u>a</u> <u>hard</u> <u>time</u> <u>losing</u> <u>weight</u> (body fat) you might be insulin resistant. It is estimated that one-third of Americans are insulin resistant (a condition also called metabolic syndrome). *Aside from difficulty losing weight, the consequences of insulin resistance include: increased body fat around the middle; physical and/or mental fatigue; sleepiness after meals; bloating and depression.* The *Eating Plans* in this book are *excellent* for people who have become insulin resistant and represent the state-of-the-art in dietary therapy. <u>The</u> <u>most</u> <u>important</u> <u>goal</u> <u>of</u> <u>any</u> <u>dietary</u> <u>program</u> <u>or</u> <u>strategy</u> <u>should</u> <u>be</u> <u>improving</u> <u>insulin</u> <u>sensitivity</u> <u>and</u> <u>controlling</u> <u>blood</u> <u>sugar</u> <u>levels.</u>

The foods (carbohydrates) you consume trigger the amount of insulin released by your pancreas gland. High levels of sugar in the bloodstream from carbohydrate foods eaten, force the pancreas to release large amounts of insulin. Insulin resistance occurs over time when our body is exposed to repeated high levels of blood sugar. Eventually, the cells in our body become accustomed to these high levels and they no longer "hear" the signal insulin gives the cell to absorb the sugar in the blood stream. At the same time, <u>the</u> <u>body</u> <u>is</u> <u>forced</u> <u>to</u> <u>store</u> <u>sugars</u> <u>as</u> <u>fat.</u>

Here's the net effect on weight loss: <u>Two</u> <u>negative</u> <u>dynamics</u> <u>occur</u> <u>as</u> <u>we</u> <u>become</u> <u>insulin</u> resistant. First, our cells become starved for sugar they need to make energy. Second, <u>we</u> <u>become</u>

fatter! *Now this is where things get really ugly.* Our body *feels hungry all the time* because our cells are not responding to insulin's command to absorb the sugar in the blood, so they become energy deprived. And since we feel hungry, we eat more food (often more carbohydrate foods we start to crave), thereby increasing our body fat. This downward spiral ends in a disease state called Type II Diabetes, a condition that increases our risk of heart attacks and virtually every known chronic disease.

Eating an overabundance of carbohydrate foods, especially the highly processed ones (covered in *"Food 101"*) and high glycemic ones (covered next) common in most American's diets, can lead to chronically elevated insulin levels and insulin resistance. High insulin levels can cause many other health problems, such as obesity, inflammatory conditions, and premature aging. They can also increase the rate of stiffness in the body, weaken joints, affect memory and cognition, and suppress the immune system.

The best way to improve insulin sensitivity and thereby stop your body from converting sugar to fat is by controlling your carbohydrate intake. Different ways of affecting this are: eating low-glycemic foods (covered next); eating alkaline vegetables; eating protein with carbohydrates; increasing fiber intake; eating smaller, more frequent meals; and blending proteins and healthy fats with carbohydrates for more *balanced* meals – all of which are incorporated in the *Eating Plans* in this section.

For many people, it is particularly helpful to use blood sugar balancing supplements, like *Carb Cheater* (recommended in the *Supplement Section*). Also, new cutting-edge research has shown that Omega-3 fish oil supplements improve insulin sensitivity ("exerting positive effects on insulin resistance in overweight individuals"). A high-potency Omega-3 supplement, *Optimal Omega HP* is also recommended in the *Supplement Section*.

Also, exercise promotes insulin sensitivity by using calories (sugar) for energy, whereas not exercising encourages insulin resistance and the storage of calories in fat cells.

7. Glycemic Index:

The glycemic index measures (or ranks) how quickly carbohydrate rich foods (fruits, vegetables, grains, sugars) raise a person's blood sugar and consequent need for insulin. A *high* ranking or value (not good) causes more rapid spikes in blood sugar and insulin. Carbohydrate foods that do this are avoided in these plans. The ones that have *low* rankings or values (good), have a lesser effect on blood sugar and insulin, and are recommended.

A newer measure called *the glycemic load* takes into account the glycemic index and how much carbohydrates are in a serving of the food. I mention it because you will be hearing this term a lot more in the future. The quantity of carbohydrates consumed is also important, and should be considered and regulated in any weight loss plan.

8. Fiber:

Dietary Fiber is simply a type or part of carbohydrates contained in foods like fruits, vegetables, and grains that cannot be digested and pass through our digestive tract intact. "Bulking up" with fiber can help people slim down.

Fiber helps promote weight loss in three ways. *First*, fiber slows down the transit time of foods in the intestinal tract, which provides a feeling of fullness that helps curb hunger cravings. *Second*, and more exciting, fiber helps reduce the number of calories absorbed from the foods we eat. *Third*, fiber also reduces the release and absorption of carbohydrates to blood sugar, thus helping to control insulin levels and the negative effects of higher glycemic foods.

The reason I consider fiber one of the best anti-aging and longevity nutrients is that it has also been shown to help improve regularity and relieve occasional constipation, relieve bloating, reduce cholesterol, maintain healthy blood pressure, reduce blood sugar swings, and relieve digestive problems.

The problem is *most people are severely deficient in fiber* – with 9 out of 10 Americans not getting the daily recommended amount (25 grams for women and 38 for men). The *Eating Plans* contain foods with higher fiber amounts, plus this is also why I recommend the use of a new, super-concentrated fiber supplement called *Ready Fiber*, that contains 12 grams of fiber in a single ounce!

9. **Hormone Imbalances and Declines:**
   Hormone imbalances and hormone declines (age-related, and lifestyle or diet induced) halt weight loss or make it very difficult, can cause weight gain, prematurely age the body, and cause many health issues that are often misdiagnosed or incorrectly treated. The following information can dramatically change your health and weight loss:

   Growth Hormone
   Growth Hormone (also referred to as HGH) is naturally produced by our bodies in abundance when we are young, but its production gradually slows over time, falling more than 75% from age 20 to 60. Unlike other hormones, Growth Hormone affects almost every body tissue. Growth Hormone is a master hormone controlling many organs and body functions and is directly responsible for stimulating tissue repair and cell replacement.

   Growth Hormone is responsible for helping the body to lose fat, build lean muscle, sleep better, improve sexual performance, increase energy and motivation, improve skin appearance and wrinkles, and much more.

   Diet and exercise (certain types – covered in the *Exercise Section*) can optimize Growth Hormone levels in the body. Also, Growth Hormone levels can significantly increase (naturally) when insulin levels are low. Therefore, the avoidance of high insulin producing and glycemic index foods is also beneficial for supporting better

"44 Year-Old Man Loses 32 Pounds And 6 Inches From His Waist!"

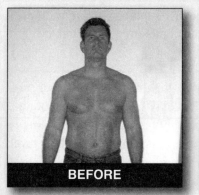

BEFORE

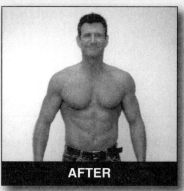

AFTER

Eating Plans

When Erick wanted to lose the pounds he had gained over the years, he said he "*didn't want to try some crazy diet fad, especially one with any unsafe stimulants.*" Erick used *Plan A* very strictly, exercised lightly with weights for "*no more than 30 minutes, three times a week,*" and used the recommended supplements, *AminoSculpt*, *Sculpt n' Cleanse*, and *Nature's Optimal Nutrition (Ready Fiber was not available then)*.

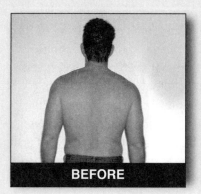

BEFORE

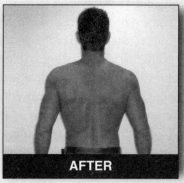

AFTER

Erick says, "*The results speak for themselves. Not only did I lose over thirty pounds of fat (my weight went from 238 to 206), but I also lost about 6 inches from my waist. Plus, Sculpt n' Cleanse helps keep me regular and I have no bloating.*" Erick also noticed, "*When using AminoSculpt my skin got softer and the tone improved. Even with all the weight lost, I didn't have any loose skin, and my skin looks years younger! I was even told I had the body and skin of an eighteen year old – and I'm 44!*"

Growth Hormone levels.

To optimize Growth Hormone levels, we need to:
1) Avoid high insulin producing and glycemic index foods (certain carbohydrates), and
2) Avoid eating food during the last 3-4 hours before bedtime, when Growth Hormone and its fat burning potential are at their peak.

The *Eating Plans* will help you to do this. Also, the use of *AminoSculpt* at bedtime (with its Growth Hormone promoting amino acids) is also recommended. Plus, in the *Exercise Section*, I'll share how to naturally increase your Growth Hormone levels with a specific type of exercise and routine.

Adrenal Fatigue

The adrenal glands produce hormones (Cortisol and DHEA included), which affect weight loss (and weight gain), immune function, energy levels, memory and mental clarity, and mood and/or feelings of well-being.

A continual exposure to *stress, poor eating habits* (especially consumption of refined carbohydrates, high glycemic foods, fried foods, sugars, and caffeine) *and/or acute chronic infections*, including digestive types (e.g. bacterial overgrowth, yeast and fungal intestinal infections, candida, food allergies, gluten sensitivities, etc.) can cause a continual overproduction of the hormone *Cortisol*, which eventually results in *adrenal fatigue* (with advanced stages leading to *adrenal exhaustion*). This is the type of fatigue sleep can't fix. Those suffering from this often have to use caffeinated beverages, like coffee and colas, and other stimulants to get through the day.

Common symptoms of adrenal fatigue include: *inability to lose weight, weight gain around the middle, fatigue, a lack of energy, constantly being tired (or feeling "burned out"), depression, sweet cravings, decreased sex drive, insomnia, memory problems, anxiety, lowered immune function (with more frequent colds and illnesses and the susceptibility to them), nervousness, irritability, insomnia, menstrual irregularities, low blood sugar, hair loss, cold feet or hands, low blood pressure and joint and/or muscle pain.* Abnormal Cortisol levels from chronic stress and adrenal fatigue can also lead to bone loss and inflammation.

In relation to weight loss, increased Cortisol levels result in weight gain (or can hamper or stop weight loss) by causing:
1) *A loss of muscle mass* (by breaking down muscles; decreasing protein synthesis; reducing tissue building hormones, e.g. DHEA, Growth Hormone, Testosterone, and others; and decreasing the metabolism).
2) *Increasing blood sugar levels* (including decreased insulin sensitivity, and increased appetite and carbohydrate cravings).
3) *Increasing body fat* (from the increased appetite and decreased metabolism) with a redistribution or accumulation of body fat in the midline or abdominal region.

Most people will experience adrenal fatigue or exhaustion at some point in their life.

If any of this sounds like you - don't worry – even simple changes to your lifestyle can help. Some of the best dietary ways to improve your adrenal health are: avoiding refined carbohydrates, high glycemic foods, sugars, caffeine or stimulants; eating foods rich in Vitamin B and C; and eating more frequent meals (which avoids low blood sugar) – all of which are incorporated in the upcoming *Eating Plans.*

A supplement that can support adrenal health is a comprehensive, high-potency multivitamin (like *Nature's Optimal Nutrition*) to ensure you receive all (and additional amounts) of the nutrients needed to support adrenal function.

Also, proper rest, the avoidance of overly stressful situations, deep breathing, meditation, yoga, light exercise, and even a quick five minute break in the middle of a hectic day can help heal your adrenal glands.

Excess Environmental Estrogens

Excess amounts of the hormone, Estrogen, from environmental sources, can cause excess fat on the waistline, hips, and thighs, as well as other health problems.

Our bodies are exposed to *"excess environmental estrogen"* from hormones fed to animals (in our meat and dairy); pesticides (on our fruits and vegetables); and from man-made estrogens, call *xenoestrogens* (in processed foods, plastics, and cosmetics). Constant exposure to these creates an excess estrogen imbalance in the body, which affects other hormones and the metabolism.

Symptoms of excess estrogen include: *weight gain; fat accumulation in the waistline, hips and thighs (especially with women); cravings for sweets and carbohydrates; blood sugar imbalances; fatigue; headaches; digestive problems; bloating; memory problems; and for women, water retention, PMS, breast pain, and menstrual problems.*

Excess estrogen affects weight gain by binding to receptors in the body's hormone-sensitive (fatty tissue) in the waistline, buttocks, hips and thighs. This conversion of body fat, and the production of more estrogen, stimulates a cycle of even more fat storage.

Once again, you can correct this imbalance and reduce the excess estrogen by controlling your diet. In some people, just this simple change can result in rapid weight loss. Ways to do this are: avoiding refined carbohydrates, sugars, sweets, artificial sweeteners, caffeine, alcohol, and processed foods like bacon and sausage; using organic foods, especially dairy (e.g. milk) and hormone-free meats; thoroughly washing fruits and vegetables to remove pesticides and/or using organic ones; eating detoxifying cruciferous vegetables (like broccoli, cauliflower), leafy greens, and fruits (like pomegranates); consuming certain fats (avocados, nuts, seeds, olives) and related oils; using certain spices (like oregano, turmeric, thyme, sage, and rosemary); incorporating certain flavorings (like lemon juice and apple cider vinegar); and drinking ample amounts of pure water.

The goal of consuming certain foods and avoiding others is to avoid consuming additional excess estrogens, while improving and supporting liver function to help process and eliminate excess estrogens already in your body. Once again, the upcoming *Eating Plans* and the accompanying food tips and guidelines help accomplish this.

Consumption of adequate amounts of fiber (including higher concentrations like in *Ready Fiber*) with meals can help absorb and eliminate excess estrogens eaten. Also, cleansing supplements (like *Sculpt n' Cleanse*) can be used to accelerate the removal of toxins and waste.

Eating Plans

When utilizing these nine fat-fighting strategies, you'll experience quick and extraordinary weight loss, body shaping, and health improvements. Combined, as in this entire program, they provide a unique and successful system to:

1. Build lean muscle tissue,
2. Cleanse and purify your body,
3. Stabilize blood sugar levels,
4. Improve digestion and your gastro-intestinal functions,
5. Balance and improve your hormone levels, and
6. Reduce inflammation.

Food 101

We've all heard the phrase, "You are what you eat." Well, the good news is there are only three types of food that you need to know about in discovering how you got where you are at, and in reshaping your body to where you want it to be.

If you have previously read anything about *Protein, Carbohydrates, and Fat* (the three types), make sure you don't skip this section as I give it my own spin for weight loss…

Protein

The word "protein" comes from the Greek word meaning "*of first importance.*" After water and oxygen, protein is one of the most prevalent and essential nutrients and structural substances in our bodies. Our muscles, organs, glands, bones, teeth, skin, hair, nails are all made up of protein. It is a constituent of every cell, and the functional element in our hormones, enzymes and glandular secretions. <u>Protein is also critical for tissue growth and repair.</u>

Proteins are made up of building blocks called *amino acids.* There are two types of amino acids: *indispensable* and *non-dispensable* (these were formerly called *essential* and *non-essential*). Indispensable amino acids cannot be made by your body and must be obtained from food. Foods that contain all the indispensable amino acids are referred to as "complete" proteins. These are animal sources of protein – meat, fish, fowl, eggs and diary products. Foods that lack all of the indispensable amino acids are called "incomplete" proteins. These are plant proteins, such as grains, beans, fruits and vegetables.

When you do not have enough protein in your diet, your body will break down your muscle tissue to meet its protein needs. When this happens during dieting, you will end up with an un-toned body and loose skin. Instead you should <u>gain muscle</u> when dieting (explained in the first section). This is why my clients and I have toned, firm and more youthful bodies (as you can see in our after pictures).

And, <u>when you diet or exercise, your body requires more protein</u> than normal. One reason for this is that when the body endures stress or trauma (injury, illness, exercise, or even dieting), the non-dispensable amino acids can become *conditionally indispensable* (meaning they must be obtained from food), due to the fact that the body may not be able to make enough to support this extra need.

This is why consuming proper amounts of protein is so important. While food is preferred as a source for protein, it cannot always be digested and assimilated well by the body. This is why it makes sense to use protein supplements. The upcoming plans, and the inclusion of supplements like *AminoSculpt*, will help you consume an adequate amount of protein to achieve a toned, firm, healthy and youthful body.

Sources of protein include: meat, fish, fowl, eggs and dairy products. Except for protein sources like seeds and nuts, an easy way to remember protein foods is that they *come from something that has "eyes,"* like cows, chickens (eggs), pigs, fish, etc.

Carbohydrates

The primary role of carbohydrates is for use by the body for energy. Although proteins and fats can be converted to energy, carbohydrates are the body's preferred source.

When carbohydrate intake is limited, and/or certain types of carbohydrates are emphasized (i.e. fibrous and complex) and others are avoided (i.e. simple or refined sugars), the body will draw upon its fat stores to provide energy – thus resulting in weight loss.

An easy way to remember carbohydrates is that they are from foods that *do not have eyes* – vegetables, fruits, and grains.

Carbohydrates are considered "refined" or "unrefined." *Unrefined* ones are carbohydrates that come from foods that have not been processed. These types are typically foods in their natural state (yams, brown rice, wheat, oats, certain vegetables). They contain many naturally occurring nutrients and usually have a lower glycemic value (good). *Refined* carbohydrates are those foods that have been processed (i.e. white flour products, breads, white rice, pasta, soda, sweets). These foods have been stripped of their naturally occurring nutrients and contain higher calories (thus they are referred to as "empty calories"). They also have a higher glycemic value and rapidly increase insulin levels (both not good).

I break carbohydrates down into three general groups: *simple* carbohydrates (sugars), *complex* carbohydrates (starches), and *fibrous* carbohydrates (fibers or fibrous). In my experience, the type of carbohydrate and amount you consume are two of the biggest factors in determining your weight loss success and how quickly your results are achieved. It is vitally important to know which foods fall in what carbohydrate categories.

Complex Carbohydrates:
Complex carbohydrates (the unrefined ones) take longer to break down and absorb so they are less likely to be stored as fat. This provides a longer energy boost and does not rapidly spike insulin levels (which is good). Complex carbohydrates contain more calories though, so even the good ones should be limited.

Good (unrefined) complex carbohydrate sources are: sweet potatoes, beans, peas, whole wheat, oatmeal, and brown rice (these are in upcoming *Eating Plan B*). Complex carbohydrates that should be avoided are refined ones, like white flour, pasta, white rice, and breads. In my *Eating Plans*, certain unrefined complex carbohydrates, like potatoes and carrots are also limited as they have a high glycemic value, thus having a greater effect on blood sugar, insulin and fat storage. As a note, most root or "under the ground" vegetables are complex carbohydrates, and have higher glycemic values (more sugar). These also contain higher amounts of carbohydrates and calories, so you'll want to limit and avoid eating them in the evening when using *Eating Plan B*.

Fibrous Carbohydrates:
Fibrous carbohydrates are like complex carbohydrates, but contain higher amounts of fiber and lower amounts of calories. They are typically "above ground" vegetables and have lower glycemic values (less sugar), which is preferable. They also usually contain more nutrients, phytonutrients, and antioxidants.

These are typically "crunchy" vegetables, like green beans, broccoli, celery, asparagus, cauliflower and salad vegetables. Because of their high fiber content, they will also satisfy your appetite making you feel full. *These are the best carbohydrates you can consume for losing weight quickly.*

Simple Carbohydrates (Sugars):

Simple carbohydrates are commonly referred to as sugars. This type of carbohydrate is absorbed directly into the blood stream and typically requires little to no digestion. They are easily converted to body fat. Most of these carbohydrates stimulate a rapid insulin response (not good). Since they are absorbed easily, they leave you feeling hungry sooner than complex or fibrous carbohydrates. They also give you short bursts of energy and bigger letdowns.

I divide these into two groups: fruits and processed sugar foods.

Fruits and Fruit Juices:

These include all types of fruits. Because most of them are higher in carbohydrates and calories, plus are easily converted to body fat, most are a poor choice and should be avoided when dieting. Certain fruits that contain lower calories, higher fiber, and/or a lower glycemic value are included. Also, certain juices used in small amounts at strategic times are also included on a very limited basis. Although you are able to get your nutrients from vegetable (fibrous and complex) carbohydrates, I recommend supplementing with a high potency multivitamin/mineral, like *Nature's Optimal Nutrition* to ensure you are getting them all.

Processed Sugars:

These include refined foods like sweets (candies, ice cream, etc), sodas, chips, snacks; as well as white sugar, brown sugar, corn syrups, most maltodextrins, dextrose, and sucrose. If there is a heaven and hell in the food kingdom, these belong in hell. They are also "empty calories" containing virtually no nutritional value, are high in calories, have high glycemic indexes, and will shoot your insulin levels through the roof, easily storing body fat.

For weight loss always choose fibrous and then unrefined complex carbohydrate foods over refined, simple or sugar, and fruit carbohydrate foods.

Fat

Dietary fats are also referred to as lipids. Fats function in the body as structural components for all cell membranes; insulation, support, and protection of your organs. Fats also serve as carriers for the fat-soluble vitamins A, D, E, and K, aiding in their absorption; and in hormone production (critical in anti-aging and weight loss).

There are two types of fat: *saturated* and *unsaturated*. Unsaturated fats are anti-sticky and more fluid. Contrary to what many people think, *both* of these fats are important for a healthy body. There are several important fatty acids the body *cannot manufacture* - these are called "essential fatty acids" (EFAs). There are two types of EFAs: Omega-3 and Omega-6. Most people should focus on consuming more Omega-3's (as they usually consume enough Omega 6's in their diets). Good sources of EFAs are fresh seeds and nuts, sprouted grains, vegetables, and cold water fish (which Omega-3 fish oils are produced from). Two of the better sources for EFAs are olive oil (a main component of the scientifically proven healthy Mediterranean diet) and Omega-3 fish oils.

Healthy fats help the body burn calories; improve insulin sensitivity; reduce inflammation; reduce the risk of heart disease; support healthy cholesterol and blood pressure levels; improve mood and feelings of well-being; support vision health, support memory and concentration, and support healthy skin, hair and nails.

Congratulations! You've just earned your first weight loss and nutrition stripes, and you are ready to start! Now that you have this background, you will better understand what you are eating and why – and you have started the process to making better long-term choices in the foods you select even after completing this program.

My Reshape Results

"Continual Improvement –
Even During The Holidays!"

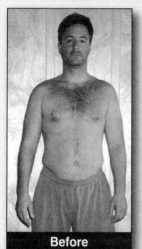
Before

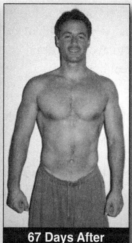
67 Days After

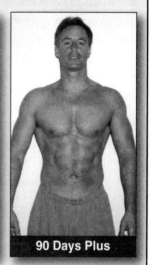
90 Days Plus

Eating Plans

If you commit to a 90 day program and follow the advice in this book, you can stay lean and in shape – and <u>improve</u> <u>your</u> <u>body</u> <u>even</u> <u>more</u>!

<u>From</u> <u>start</u> <u>to</u> <u>90</u> <u>days</u> I lost over 19 pounds of <u>fat</u>, 4 inches from my waist, 13 TOTAL inches from all over, <u>gained</u> <u>muscle</u> (which usually doesn't happen on most diets), reshaped and toned my body! Now consider this...

<u>The</u> <u>next</u> <u>6</u> <u>months</u> took me through winter and the holidays, which is when most people usually eat more and gain weight. During this time I also had two injuries (my lower back and shoulder), which limited what I could do and prevented me from exercising for a period of time.

After all that, the picture on the far right continues to show results – and I wasn't even dieting strictly! By the way, this picture was taken almost immediately after a vacation where I *definitely* wasn't dieting. *The point is once you've reached your ideal shape on this program you can easily maintain and improve upon it.*

Notice the increased development of my waist (abdominals), and the additional muscle and definition of my shoulders, chest, and arms (which was my goal) – <u>and</u> I did not gain any fat!

The Eating Plans

The following *Eating Plans* are designed to help you: 1) lose fat, 2) build and shape your body, 3) improve your health and energy levels, 4) improve your metabolism, 5) restore your body's ability to process certain foods that cause you problems, and 6) to ultimately educate you on what foods to avoid, or limit for long-term weight management and general health.

There are two weight loss eating plans (*Plans A and B*). They are designed to be flexible; this allows you to choose the one that best suits you and your lifestyle.

The Difference Between *Plan A* and *Plan B*:

In a moment you will see *Plan A* and *Plan B*. Although they look similar, the difference is that *Plan B* includes certain complex (starch) carbohydrates. These are some of the foods from the *Avoid* list in *Plan A* that have been moved to the *Limited* category.

The complex carbohydrates I recommend have a lower glycemic value and will not rapidly convert to sugar (and overly affect your insulin). They have been included since your body will be better able to control, digest and process these types of "unrefined" carbohydrates at this point.

For the Best and Quickest Results...

Ideally, start on *Eating Plan A* and move to *Eating Plan B* when indicated (*see the following timeline*). Stay on *Eating Plan B* until you complete a full 90 days (total time on both programs).

TIMELINES FOR USING *PLAN A* AND *PLAN B*	
Plan A:	Use for 3-12 weeks and then switch to *Plan B*
Plan B:	I. If you switch here from *Plan A*, then continue this for the remainder of the 90 days or until your desired weight is reached II. If you start here, use this plan for 90 days or until your desired weight is reached.

How Long On Each Plan?

For an average individual with **under 10 pounds** to lose or those who don't want to lose weight but want to redistribute it, firm up, or tone up – stay on *Plan A* for 3-4 weeks, then switch to *Plan B*.

If you need to lose over 10 pounds **or** have (or you think you have) a problem with Candida albicans, then stay on *Plan A* for 6-12 weeks. If for whatever reason you cannot do this for 6 weeks, at least give it a shot for 3 weeks as it will help prime and then turbocharge your system for fat loss and reshaping.

If you need to lose **over 40 pounds**, please understand that you can only healthily lose a certain amount of weight in a given period of time. You will show significant results in 90 days, but take 3-4 weeks off and then complete another 90 day cycle of *Plan A and B* – preferably including the recommended supplements until you reach your ideal weight.

IMPORTANT NOTE:

Anyone with a significant amount of weight to lose or anyone using this plan for longer than 90 days should be under the care and supervision of a medical professional. Anyone with any medical conditions should always consult their physician when starting this or any weight loss program.

Do This Program For 90 Days...

Although most of you will achieve your desired results in less than 90 days (like I did), this is the basic amount of time I have found it takes to have a significant change on most people's digestive systems and metabolisms. This will allow you to continue to enjoy many foods, as well as lessen the possibility of gaining weight back. Although I lost my weight in a little over 60 days, I stayed on the program for a full 90 days for this reason.

The goal is to return you to a normal, well balanced diet as soon as your body allows it. The closer you follow these eating programs, the sooner your body will respond.

The following is a summary of when and how much to take of the supplements recommended in this book in coordination with the *Eating Plans*. In a perfect world you'd take all these supplements in Levels 1 and 2. However, in the reality of living on a budget, you'll pick the most important ones. If you have to choose which ones to take, they are listed by level of importance (and within their level they are also listed in the order of importance). A summary of their purposes and benefits is on page 71, and expanded details of each follows in the *Supplement Section.*

LEVEL 1		
SUPPLEMENT	**TIMING**	**DOSE**
Sculpt n' Cleanse	✓ **In-Between Meals** on an empty stomach	1 or more capsules, once or twice a day
AminoSculpt	✓ **Bedtime,** preferably on an empty stomach	1-2 tablespoons with 8 ounces of water
Ready Fiber	✓ **Breakfast** and **Dinner**	1/2 ounce
LEVEL 2		
Nature's Optimal Nutrition	✓ **Breakfast** ✓ **Anytime when energy is needed**	1 ounce with water 1 ounce with 12 ounces of water
Optimal Omega HP	✓ **Breakfast** and **Dinner**	1-2 softgels
Protein Shake – Meal Replacement	✓ Replace **any meal** with it	25-40 grams
LEVEL 3		
Carb Cheater	✓ **With any meal** containing carbohydrates, cheat meals, or alcohol	1-3 caplets with water (preferably before eating)
Binge Buster	✓ **Any time** you have hunger or cravings	2 sprays up to 4 times per day before meals or when needed
MSM	✓ **Breakfast** and **Dinner,** or any meal	2 or more capsules

Construct your meals by choosing foods from the upcoming *Food Choices* chart and incorporate any additional nutrition tips that are mentioned. A sample menu of what your daily meals should look like also follows (under *Sample Daily Meals*).

It is very simple, you will eat as much as you want of certain foods (*Unlimited*), moderate or lesser amounts of others (*Limited and Very Limited*), and you will avoid some foods altogether (*Avoid*).

I highly recommend you have a *Protein-Meal Replacement Shake* for one or more of your meals. This is up to you. These meals are quick, convenient, tasty, and provide you with one of the best sources of readily available and absorbable protein. I've included some delicious recipes for these "shakes."

An "Off Day" and "Cheat Meal"...

On *Plan A*, two days during the week are *Off Days*. These days, you will switch to *Plan B* foods and include some complex carbohydrates that are normally restricted on *Plan A*.

Part of your *Off Days* can include a *Cheat Meal*. For one meal on this day - eat whatever you want - but within reason. During these meals, you should **not eat just to eat**. You should eat to **enjoy** a few foods that you have avoided and to **reward** yourself.

Turbocharge Your Fat Loss

To rapidly accelerate your metabolism and fat loss, you can modify the first week (only) as follows:

- For the first seven (7) days, use strict *Plan A* days with no *Off Days* or *Cheat Meals*.
- Avoid fruits and fruit juices you would use in your Protein-Shakes (if you include them). Flavor your shakes with extracts and cinnamon. Thicken by adding ice cubes. And add *Ready*

Fiber to increase feelings of fullness and fiber content.

- Make the *eighth day* a *Plan B* day, consuming the approved *complex* carbohydrates at breakfast and lunch only.
- Then continue on a regular *Plan A* week (chart shown next) for the rest of the program (or until you transition to *Plan B*).
- Make sure you consume a lot of water (amounts discussed in this section) during this week. Also, if you are including *AminoSculpt*, take it at bedtime with water.

_____

The following *Plan A* weekly schedule should work great for most people. Once again, a <u>normal *Plan A* week</u> includes two *Off Days* (which are *Plan B* days) and a *Cheat Meal* (optional). Your *Off Days* help you get through the week and stimulate your metabolism and your *Cheat Meals* reward you and let you loosen up on the weekends when most people socialize:

Eating Plan A The "Optimum" Fat Reducing Program						
Sunday	Monday	Tuesday	Wednesday	Thursday	Friday	Saturday
Regular *Plan A* Day	Regular *Plan A* Day	Regular *Plan A* Day	(OFF DAY) *Plan B* Day	Regular *Plan A* Day	Regular *Plan A* Day	(OFF DAY) *Plan B* Day and *Cheat Meal*

<u>Notes</u>:

Timing: You can have your *Off Day* and *Cheat Meal* on any day you like, but <u>try to keep them 3 days apart</u> **<u>or</u>** <u>only have them once a week on the same day</u>.

Off Day: Include the following complex carbohydrate foods from *Plan B* in your <u>daytime</u> meals (try to avoid them at dinner) if you want: oatmeal, sweet potato, yam, brown rice, sprouted flourless bread, beans (without lard), and an occasional white potato.

If You Are Not Taking Sculpt n' Cleanse: I would highly

recommend <u>not</u> having a *Cheat Meal*, and limiting your *Off Days* to half a day (the earlier hours).

If You Have Candida: Then it would be wise to eliminate the *Off Day* and the *Cheat Meal* as these foods are normally restricted on Candida diets.

Eating Plan B

A weekly schedule for *Plan B* is simply every day being a *Plan B* day with a *Cheat Meal* (optional) being on any day once a week. Additional details on a *Plan B* day are in the upcoming *Eating Plan Guidelines*.

What To Notice On The Cheat Days...

You will eventually notice that your *Cheat Meal* <u>does</u> <u>not</u> <u>make</u> <u>you</u> <u>feel</u> <u>good</u> <u>at</u> <u>all</u>. Some people even feel "off," fatigued, or even get a headache for a day or two after this meal (especially if you have desserts, ice cream, alcohol, or greasy foods).

This is because as you clean out your body and restore your health, your body will negatively react to bad or unhealthy foods. The reason you may not have noticed this before is because your body has been conditioned to not feeling well (<u>you</u> <u>probably</u> <u>feel</u> <u>this</u> <u>way</u> <u>most</u> <u>of</u> <u>the</u> <u>time</u> <u>and</u> <u>do</u> <u>not</u> <u>really</u> <u>notice</u> <u>it</u>). For example, do you run out of energy in the afternoons, or do you feel sluggish getting up in the morning? Most people have accepted this as normal, and it is not.

Bye-Bye Cravings...

Certain foods (the bad ones - most of the ones on the *Plan B Avoid List*) <u>are</u> <u>addicting</u>. It is normal for you to crave some of these foods when you first start a "clean" eating program like this. The good news is that usually after 3-7 days, your cravings will subside and you will not want these foods at all. If you want extra help to eliminate cravings quickly, I recommend a supplement, *Binge Buster,* in the *Supplement Section*.

General Guidlines

- Eat 4-6 times per day spaced two to three hours apart.
- A *Protein Shake* is considered a meal. Your budget permitting, substitute these for 1-2 meals.
- Have a *protein* source at every meal.
- Have 1-2 *fibrous carbohydrate* sources at every meal.
- Avoid having any food two, preferably three hours *before* bedtime (with the exception of *AminoSculpt*).
- On strict *Plan A* days, you can add a serving of nuts, nut butter, cheeses, or avocado to your meals or for snacks. And occasionally one piece of sprouted, flourless bread with a protein shake.
- If you are one of the rare people whose body has a harder time without complex/starch carbohydrates, on *Plan A* days include an approved complex/starch carbohydrate from the *Food Choices*. *Limit it to once a day before 3:00 p.m.* and try to get to where you can do without it.
- Try to have your largest meal at breakfast, and a modest or your smallest meal at dinner.

Additional Guidlines When On *Plan B*

- Have a *complex carbohydrate* source two-three times daily, and…
- Avoid having *complex carbohydrates* in your meals *after* 3:00 p.m.
- Your budget permitting, use *Carb Cheater* with meals containing complex carbohydrates.

Beverages

- Have a <u>minimum</u> of 8 glasses of water per day (preferably distilled or filtered - as pure a source as possible).
- Use Green Tea (moderately) in place of coffee or regular teas (avoid these as much as possible). Green Tea has many health benefits, and can help inhibit carbohydrate absorption and burn calories.

Exercise Meals

- If you exercise first thing in the morning, do so on an empty stomach (exception: you can take a serving of *AminoSculpt*).

- If you exercise later in the day, avoid having complex carbohydrates in the meal *before*. You can take another serving of *Nature's Optimal Nutrition prior* to exercise for increased energy (but not before the morning workout).

- After exercise, immediately have a *post exercise shake* (detailed in the shake recipes part of this section) <u>within</u> 60 minutes.

Sample Daily Meals

Eating Plan A

Breakfast
Eggs
Bell Pepper
Tomato
(make omelet)

Morning Snack
Celery
Nuts or Nut Butter

Lunch
Tuna
Salad
Broccoli

Afternoon Snack
Protein Shake

Dinner
Chicken Breast
Green Beans
Tomato, Cucumber Salad

Eating Plan B

Breakfast
Eggs
Oatmeal

Morning Snack
Cottage Cheese
Fresh Berries

Lunch
Turkey Breast
Brown Rice
Green Beans

Afternoon Snack
Hard Boiled Egg(s)
Celery

Dinner
Salmon
Salad
Asparagus

Eating Plans

Food Choices

Plan A & B	Plan A & B	Plan B Only
Proteins	**Fibrous Carbohydrates/ Vegetables**	**Complex/Starch Carbohydrates**

Unlimited

Proteins	Fibrous Carbohydrates/Vegetables	Complex/Starch Carbohydrates

Chicken Breast
Turkey Breast
Lean Ground
  Turkey
Fish
Lean Beef
Veal
Elk
Buffalo
Venison
Ostrich
Eggs*
Protein Powders*
AminoSculpt
	All Green Vegetables
	Broccoli
	Cabbage
	Green Beans
	Asparagus
	Cauliflower
	Celery
	Cucumbers
	Onions
	Lettuce
	Spinach
	Bell Peppers
	  (All Types)
	Brussel Sprouts
	Radishes
		Oatmeal
		Sweet Potatoes
		Yams
		Brown Rice
		Beans
		Corn
		Squash
		Pumpkin
		Peas

Limited

Proteins	Fibrous Carbohydrates/Vegetables	Complex/Starch Carbohydrates

Skinless Dark
  Meat Chicken
Skinless Dark
  Meat Turkey
Canned Tuna Fish
Lean Ground Beef
Pork (lean cuts-
  chops)
Lamb (lean cuts)
Shellfish
Low-fat Cottage
  Cheese*
Low or Reduced
  Fat Dairy*
Yogurt*
Soy/Tofu
Nuts
	Tomatoes
	Mushrooms
	Avocados
	Artichokes
		White Potato
		  (baked)
		Sprouted,
		  Flourless Bread
		Whole Wheat
		  Products*
		Cream of Rice
		Popcorn (no butter
		  or salt)
		Carrots

Plan A & B	Plan A & B	Plan B Only
Proteins	Fibrous Carbohydrates/ Vegetables	Complex/Starch Carbohydrates

Avoid Processed Meats
Deli/Lunch Meats
Bacon
Ham
Sausage
Non-Fat Dairy
Peanuts
		Processed
		   Carbohydrates
		White Flour
		   Products
		Pasta
		White Rice
		Cereals
		Breads
		Rice Cakes

Notes: See the notes below in the *"Very Limited"* section and the *"In the Kitchen Basics And Food Notes"* section.

Also Avoid

All Refined Carbohydrates, Sugars, Alcohol, Foods with Chemicals or Preservatives, Junk and Fast Foods, Artificial Sweeteners, Honey, Caffeinated Beverages, Soda/Soft Drinks (including diet ones), Canned Foods, Margarine, Fried Foods, Salted Products, Protein Bars, Sports Drinks (i.e. Gatorade®, vitamin waters, etc), all Energy Drinks (Rock Star®, Red Bull®, etc.), Concentrated Fruit Juices, Orange Colored Cheeses, Regular Mayonnaise, Dried Fruits, Sweets, Candies, Catsup, Grapes.

Very Limited

Fruits: Apples, Berries (Strawberry, Blueberry, Boysenberry – the darker ones are the best), Grapefruit, Bananas and Fresh Fruit Juices (only in small amounts with your protein shakes). *Condiments:* Mayonnaise (non-hydrogenated). *Nuts:* Cashews, Almonds, Brazil Nuts, or Walnuts. *Cheeses:* Raw and uncolored, Feta cheese. *Dairy:* Dairy and Milk Products – Preferably raw and organic. Also use low or reduced fat (limit whole, avoid non-fat ones). With yogurts, only plain, no added fruit yogurts.

Eating Plans

- *Portion Sizes:* An easy way to measure foods is to use your hand to approximate portion sizes. Protein portions can be the size of your *open palm*, and vegetable and complex carbohydrate portions can be the size of your *closed fist*.

- *Cooking:* Broil, bake, or boil – DO NOT FRY.

On all the following foods (where applicable, e.g. fruits, vegetables, meats, eggs, and any others) do your best (and budget permitting) to buy organic, raw and/or free-range products.

- *Alcohol:* These are on the avoid list, but if you are going to indulge, stay with dry red wine (best), and light and low-carb beers. Eat protein and fats (i.e. cheese and nuts) with alcohol to reduce its effect on increasing blood sugar and insulin. Take *Carb Cheater* before to help reduce some of the negative effects of the carbohydrates. *MSM* will help also.

- *Eggs:* You can have whole eggs, egg whites, or a mixture of both. Avoid imitation eggs (Egg Beaters®, etc.). Use organic and/or cage-free (free-range) eggs whenever possible.

- *Fish:* Consume wild and avoid farmed fish.

- *Fruits:* Consume approved fruits on a very limited basis; typically as snacks or in your protein shakes.

- *Meats and Fowl:* Most importantly, try to buy *hormone and antibiotic free* meats whenever possible. Hormone laden meats can prevent weight loss and cause other health challenges. Also, organic and grass-fed meats are preferred, if available.

- *Meats (Red):* Red meats contain special forms and combinations of amino acids that are essential to the human body and are not biologically comparable to amino acids found in other protein sources or vegetables. *On this eating program try to include at least 9 oz. of red meat per week.* Red meats include beef, lamb, ostrich, buffalo, venison, reindeer, etc. **IF YOU DO NOT EAT RED MEATS**, you can obtain these special amino acids in the supplement, *AminoSculpt*. Make sure you include its use.

- *Nuts:* Eat raw nuts and nut butters. Avoid roasted and/or salted nuts and butters. Cashews, almonds, walnuts, and brazil nuts are good. Avoid peanuts as some people are allergic to these. Soaking nuts and seeds for 12-24 hours before eating is helpful for digestion whenever possible.

- *Oils:* Use olive oil on vegetables for seasoning (with lemon), on salad dressings, or for cooking. Butter, coconut oil and palm oil are good for cooking. Flaxseed oil is also good, but not for cooking. Avoid Trans-Fatty Acids and hydrogenated oils.

- *Protein Powders:* Use protein powders that: 1) do not not contain artificial sweeteners, like aspartame, sucralose, and acesulfame K; and 2) contain a very low amount of carbohydrates per serving. Do not use soy proteins. See the upcoming *Protein Shake – Meal Replacement* recommendation page in this section for further details.

- *Salt:* Limit salts. No regular refined salts; use Sea Salt or preferably Celtic Sea Salt.

- *Seasonings/Other:* Oregano, rosemary and garlic are very good. Curry, cumin, ginger, sage, thyme, and turmeric can also help *flush* excess estrogen from the body.

- *Snacks:* Some quick snack ideas are: *half an apple with nut butter or a handful or nuts, celery and tuna, celery and nut butter, yogurt and berries, hard boiled eggs alone or with fibrous vegetables.* Keep in mind these are limited, meaning once a day or a few times per week, if you are really strict.

- *Sweeteners:* No artificial sweeteners. Stevia is fine. Cinnamon is good as it helps balance blood sugar levels.

- *Vegetables:* Fresh or frozen (not canned or pre-cooked). Prepared raw, or steamed is best. Lightly grilled is fine. Avoid overcooking. Limit avocado use to one half per day (good for hormone balancing). Organic is preferred.

Eating Plans

- *Vinegar:* Preferably use apple cider vinegar for salad dressings and with foods (it has many reported benefits and I have found it reduces the appetite).

- *Water:* Adequate water consumption reduces hunger, accelerates weight loss, improves energy levels, and is needed when cleansing to flush toxins (including excess estrogens) out of the body. A good rule is to drink half of your body weight in ounces of water per day (for most people this is between 64 and 128 ounces). Avoid chlorinated and tap water (which can have high levels of contaminants). Drink filtered or distilled waters.

  The best and purest water available I have found is a brand called *Pure Inspiration*. It has a PH of 8.6 (very high which is good), low surface tension, a positive polarity - all of which are important in cleansing the cells and flushing toxins from the body. This water and its extraordinary healthy features are naturally occurring with no man-made enhancements or processing (unlike many other "health" waters available). You can find *Pure Inspiration* by going to: **www.PureInspirationWater.com**

- *Wheat and Grains:* If you can, avoid glutens (wheat, rye and barley) products. Good substitutes are rice, corn, amaranth, buckwheat, flax, millet, and quinoa. For more information on what foods contain glutens, go to **www.celiac.org**, or **www.gluten.org**

Tasty *Plan A* and *Plan B* Meal Recipes

A holistic nutritionist and organic chef friend of mine, Brigitte Malaaya Britton (author of *The Mega Way*) has created a number of gourmet recipes that you can use on *Plan B*, and some for *Plan A*. I have also compiled meal recipes that my clients and I have used. Simply go to: **www.reshapeforlife.com** for all these and other resources that will assist you on this program.

Protein – Meal Replacement Shake Recipes

The following are delicious shake recipes that I've discovered over the years, or ones that have been submitted by my clients. Enjoy!

Basic Vanilla
- 25-30 gms Vanilla Protein Powder
- 6 oz. Water
- 4-6 Ice Cubes

Basic Chocolate
- 25-30 gms Chocolate Protein Powder
- 6 oz. Water
- 4-6 Ice Cubes

Apple Strawberry
- 25-30 gms Vanilla Protein Powder
- 2-4 oz. Apple Juice
- 4 oz. Water
- 4-5 Frozen Strawberries

Chocolate Truffle
- 25-30 gms Chocolate Protein Powder
- 2-4 oz. Pomegranate Juice
- 4 oz. Water
- 3-4 Frozen Strawberries

Apple Banana
- 25-30 gms Vanilla Protein Powder
- 2-4 oz. Apple Juice
- 4 oz. Water
- ½ Banana

Chocolate Almond
- 25-30 gms Chocolate Protein Powder
- 8 oz. Water
- ½ Banana
- Almond Extract (4 drops)

Strawberry Supreme
- 25-30 gms Vanilla Protein Powder
- 6 oz. Water
- 1 cup Frozen Strawberries
- 2 Ice Cubes

Curt's Blender Dream
- 20-25 gms Vanilla Protein Powder
- 3 oz. Water
- 2-4 oz. Apple Juice
- 1 cup Plain Yogurt
- 5-7 Frozen Strawberries

Post Exercise Shakes

The following shakes have higher <u>acceptable</u> carbohydrate amounts (and some very limited ones) included, as this is beneficial when taken <u>only</u> and *immediately after <u>taxing</u> exercise.*

Chocolate Berry
- 30 gms Chocolate Protein Powder*
- 8 oz. Pomegranate Juice
- 2-3 Frozen Strawberries
- 2 Ice Cubes

Strawberry Banana
- 30 gms Vanilla Protein Powder*
- 8 -10 oz. Water
- 1 Whole Banana
- 5-7 Frozen Strawberries
- 2 Ice Cubes

Note: For men, 40 grams

Protein Shake Notes

<u>Follow</u> <u>these</u> <u>guidelines</u> <u>when</u> <u>making</u> <u>protein</u> <u>shakes</u>:

Juices: It is OK to use <u>limited</u> <u>amounts</u> of juices with your shakes. Make sure to measure the exact amount. Limit or avoid using juices with citric acid (orange, pineapple, lime, grapefruit) with protein powders.

Fruit: Use the recommended fruits in the recommended amounts. Limit the use of a banana in a shake to no more than once a day (preferably use it every other day – and especially on your *Off Day*). With frozen strawberries and fruits, make sure you get the type with no added sugar. Experiment with adding other berries, e.g., blueberries, boysenberries, raspberries, etc.

Extracts: Get your extracts (almond, vanilla, cherry, mint, etc.) without any added sugar or alcohol. You can usually find these in health food stores.

Sweeteners: Use Stevia and cinnamon to sweeten or enhance taste.

Strict Candida Diet: If you have Candida, or are following a strict diet, then avoid using fruits and fruit juices.

Other Tips When Making Your Shakes...

Fiber: Add ½ - 1 ounce of *Ready Fiber* to your shakes. This will help prolong feelings of fullness and increase your absorption of protein and nutrients.

Straight Protein: You don't have to mix other items with your protein. If you like the taste, you can just stir it with water or blend it with water and ice cubes. If you do this, add ½ - 1 ounce of *Ready Fiber* for previously mentioned reasons.

How To Choose A High Quality Protein/Meal Replacememt Supplement

In my opinion, this is one of the toughest categories to find a quality and healthy supplement. In an effort to provide a good tasting and affordable product, many supplement companies use cheaper ingredients, unhealthy sweeteners, and too many carbohydrates. There have only been a handful of products that I would even consider using over the years.

For buying a protein powder or meal replacement, I will provide basic guidelines on what to look for in purchasing these:

Protein Type:
The protein used should preferably be a milk protein (whey and/or casein), because of its anabolic (muscle building and preserving qualities), whey proteins can also support immune function. It should be low in lactose (the label term, which also includes ones that have very little to no lactose; these are usually well tolerated by those who are lactose intolerant). I do not recommend straight soy or non-animal proteins (unless you are a vegetarian) as they have inferior amino acid (protein) structures that are not as efficient for muscle preservation and development. Egg white protein is a good source if you do not use whey protein.

The type of protein *source* used will also greatly affect quality (i.e. Whey "isolates" are the highest grade – with Whey "concentrates" being the next level of quality). The better ones are going to cost more. Be wary of those huge jugs, or sacks of protein that are available at a super low price – they usually contain a low grade protein; or may use inferior processing so the bioavailability is less (meaning you have to consume a lot more to equal what you'd absorb in a smaller quantity of a higher quality one). Many companies mix or combine proteins, which is fine (and can be done for a specific purposes). The problem for consumers is being able to recognize when cheaper grades of protein are combined to lower costs.

Carbohydrate Content:
Straight proteins should have very little carbohydrate content (less than 5 grams per serving). Meal replacements should have less than 20 grams of carbohydrates (and preferably lower). If you have Candida or are sensitive to carbohydrates (even with minor insulin resistance) avoid these. Also, when on *Plan A* days, definitely do not use these. When using a meal replacement powder, take it with water, and do <u>not</u> use the shake recipes in this book, as you would consume too many carbohydrates.

As a note, maltodextrin is a commonly used carbohydrate source in many proteins and meal replacements. Since the grade of maltodextrin used can vary greatly (and you will probably not know what it is), I would avoid these.

Sweeteners:
<u>Do</u> <u>NOT</u> <u>use</u> <u>any</u> <u>proteins</u> <u>that</u> <u>contain</u> <u>artificial</u> <u>sweeteners</u> – especially *Aspartame, Sucralose (Splenda), and Acesulfame-k.* Other sweeteners to avoid are refined sugars, sucrose, dextrose, glucose, high fructose corn syrups (low amounts of regular, low glycemic fructoses are fine), brown sugars, cane sugar, evaporated cane juice, processed honey and molasses. *Acceptable sweeteners are: Stevia, Lo Han, and small amounts of fructose.*

Follow the previous guidelines to find the best quality and priced protein to suit your needs. I have also recommended a protein I use in the *Supplement Section.*

Supplements

The statements about the products discussed in this book have not been evaluated by the Food and Drug Administration. These products are not intended to diagnose, treat, cure or prevent any disease.

Pregnant women, nursing mothers or those on any medication should always consult with their health professional before using any nutritional supplement.

"How To Turbocharge Your Body And Results..."

You are taking a trip from Los Angeles to Las Vegas. It's about 300 miles and most of the road runs through hot, barren desert. You have a choice: *Would you rather drive in a new air-conditioned car or would you rather walk?*

Nutritional supplements make your experience and results much easier when dieting or on any health improvement program. I purposely use this analogy to encourage any first-timers to consider including nutritional supplements with their health improvement programs.

I am not talking about the "super-duper miracle" pill of the week or stimulants (which most fat burning and weight loss products contain). I am referring to time-tested, <u>clinically</u> <u>substantiated</u>, safe supplements that *work with your body* to naturally improve its efficiency and help restore imbalances and deficiencies.

Science has come a long way in providing efficacious, legitimate, natural, and safe weight loss aids. *Not using certain supplements for weight loss is like walking to Las Vegas - it can take a <u>lot</u> <u>longer</u> and it can be a <u>miserable</u> <u>trip</u>.*

Not taking supplements to cleanse your colon and fight Candida is like trying to walk to Las Vegas on your hands - you are going to fall over a lot and probably not make it - and if you did, it would be a long, ugly, blistering trip.

<u>Using</u> <u>supplements</u> for fat loss, <u>colon</u> <u>cleansing</u>, fighting Candida, and improving health problems is like taking the <u>air-conditioned</u> <u>car</u> - your ride is going to be as comfortable as possible and you will get there as quickly as possible. *More importantly, supplements can help give you some immediate, noticeable improvements <u>to</u> <u>keep</u> <u>you</u> <u>motivated</u> <u>and</u> <u>in</u> <u>the</u> <u>game</u> <u>so</u> <u>you</u> <u>are</u> <u>successful</u>.*

Supplements

Who Said You Don't Need Supplements?

Anyone who tells you that you do not need supplements is either living in the dark ages, trying to sell a commercial program for the masses, or just has not done their research and homework.

Be suspicious of any health professional who tells you that it is unnecessary to supplement as, "Everything you need is in food" - especially when there is overwhelming evidence that the nutrients in our food supply have continually been depleted over the last 50 years.

I am strongly opinionated here as I've personally witnessed thousands of people positively affecting their weight loss, overall health and completely turning their lives around with supplementation.

In my condition, I would have had a hard time achieving my results if I did not have some of the supplements that you are about to review.

The successful results of myself and hundreds of thousands of my clients speak for themselves. Please enjoy and utilize this shortcut...

OK, How Can I Tell What Supplements Are The Best?

This one is not that easy. You need to have a decent understanding of how the body works, some knowledge about specific nutrients (label claims are not always what you get or want), some connections in the industry can really help, and just plain trial and error which will cost you a lot of money, take a lot of time – and will probably give you a lot of gas!

Let me just start by telling you that there is a lot of garbage out there! It nauseates and infuriates me to see some of the products and claims that are made by some nutritional companies. It took me twenty-plus years and a lot of wasted money to learn what worked and what didn't. What I am about to share with you is the accumulation of my personal experience, countless hours of research, consultations with top industry and medical professionals, and good old trial and error...

Recommended Supplements

I've organized the recommended products in this section into four categories:

1. The PRIMARY Three
2. SECONDARY Supporting Products
3. The BASICS
4. PROTEIN SHAKES (Meal Replacement Powders)

1. The PRIMARY Three

"The PRIMARY Three" are the best products available and most natural to your body for weight loss, body shaping and general health.

These products are highly recommended for the best and quickest results possible.

If you have any budgetary constraints, these products should be chosen first.   They are also placed in order of importance - so choose them in this order if you cannot get them all:

1. Sculpt n' Cleanse   2. AminoSculpt   3. Ready Fiber

2. SECONDARY Supporting Products

The best sports teams usually win because they have a good second team (these products) that can come off the bench and support the first team (The PRIMARY Three).

That is where these supporting products come in. Pick and choose from them based upon your needs. You may find that you want to immediately include several.

3. The BASICS

These are "foundational" nutritional supplements everyone should take. They provide the basic nutrients your body needs to live – they are your own "insurance policy" for life. They are the best quality and the most comprehensive products available of their kind.

4. PROTEIN SHAKES (Meal Replacement Powders)

These are just as the title states. Quality products for protein supplementation and muscle preservation are important. There are a lot of low quality losers with ingredients you don't want to take in the marketplace, so at least familiarize yourself with what to avoid.

Summary Of My Recommendations

The following is a summary of the " ideal" combination of supplements I would take (and still do in maintenance amounts). *Remember this is an "ideal" recommendation and is not necessary to be successful in losing weight on this program.* It is for the many people who have asked me about the quickest and fastest way to reshape their body and improve their overall health – if they had no budgetary constraints.

Another reason I like these products is that they have a lot of additional health benefits that most other weight loss products don't have. The following supplement recommendations are based on my experience, knowledge, and results:

Use Category		Product	Primary Weight Loss Purpose	Additional Health Benefits
Weight Loss, Body Shaping, Anti-Aging	Primary	*Sculpt n' Cleanse*	✓ Cleansing ✓ Waistline reduction	Relief from bloating, occasional constipation, and relief from the effects of toxins in the body.
		AminoSculpt	✓ Fat loss ✓ Muscle promotion ✓ Metabolism improvement ✓ Body firming and toning.	Naturally increase energy levels; promote younger looking skin, hair, and nails; support healthy joint function; promote better sleep.

Use Category		Product	Primary Weight Loss Purpose	Additional Health Benefits
Weight Loss, Body Shaping, Anti-Aging	Primary	*Ready Fiber*	✓ Decreased calorie absorption ✓ Appetite satiety ✓ Blood sugar support	Supports healthy intestinal regularity and microflora; digestive support; supports healthy cholesterol and blood pressure within normal levels.
	Secondary	*Carb Cheater*	✓ Blood sugar and insulin support	Healthy cholesterol within normal levels.
		Protein Shake	✓ Protein support ✓ Muscle tone and firmness	General nutrition, immune support.
Foundational and Anti-Aging	The Basics*	*Nature's Optimal Nutrition*	✓ Complete nutritional support	Energy, immune support, heart health.
		Optimal Omega HP	✓ Complete nutritional support ✓ Weight loss support ✓ Improved insulin sensitivity	Healthy cholesterol and blood pressure within normal levels; improved inflammation response; supports joint mobility; improved hair, skin, and nails; improved vision and eye health.
Special Support	Secondary	*Binge Buster*	✓ Appetite control ✓ Metabolism support	
		MSM	✓ Candida support	Supports joint health, energy levels, digestive health, protein structure, immune function, and healthy hair, skin, and nails.

Supplements

*Note: I also include *Ready Fiber* here as a Foundational product.

Sculpt n' Cleanse®

"The #1 Rated Colon Cleansing Weight Loss Supplement"

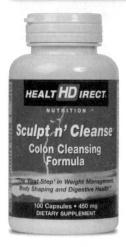

Cleansing can help*:

- Support weight loss programs
- Flatten the waistline
- Relieve occasional constipation
- Relieve bloating

Other Benefits of Cleansing:

Cleansing helps rid the body of built-up matter and toxins, which can contribute to wrinkling and skin ailments, including acne and rashes; cramping and fatigue; stiffness in joints; lack of mental clarity; as well as sinus problems, a weakened immune system, digestive problems and many other health problems.

Product Description

S*culpt n' Cleanse* is the most effective colon cleansing formula available. Cleansing should be "the first step" in any weight loss, body shaping, and general or digestive health program. Every day we are exposed to and ingest preservatives, toxins, chemicals and pollutants. In fact, typical, everyday foods and beverages that we consume, like bread, pasta, pizza, white rice, any food containing white flour; mucus forming foods like in some dairy products; sugar and alcohol products; and even fruits and vegetables are exposed to pesticides and other chemicals that can cause our bodies many health problems.

Our problem is that the body cannot properly digest and eliminate some of these foods and the substances they contain – and they can become lodged or stuck in the lining of our intestinal track in the form of old dried fecal matter and mucus. **It is estimated that** the **average person can have between 4-20 pounds of this "built-up" toxic intestinal matter in their colon** – and it can just keep accumulating over the years!

The most effective way to eliminate this toxic intestinal "build-up" is to use an herbal cleansing supplement and follow a healthy eating program, like the one recommended in this book.

Why *Sculpt n' Cleanse* is different:

- **Gentle and Safe:** It gently and safely eliminates toxic build up without causing cramping or sudden urges to evacuate.

- **Self Regulating:** It has a self regulating formula – you only take as much as your body needs.

- **Weight-Loss Results:** Additional and superior weight loss results compared to other colon cleansing supplements.

- **Cost-Effective:** The potency is greater on a per capsule basis, resulting in one bottle of *Sculpt n' Cleanse* being equivalent to 2-4 bottles of other colon cleansing products.

How to use *Sculpt n' Cleanse*:

Always use on an empty stomach preferably 30-45 minutes before meals or at least 2 hours after meals with at least one full glass of water (not juice or any other liquids). Make sure to *drink at least 8-12 glasses of water during the day when cleansing.* Start at a lower dosage and gradually work your way up.

Determining Dosage:

This is a self-regulating formula. Everyone will use different amounts, so adjust your dosage until you have *at least 2-4 bowel movements* per day. You can spread the dosage out so you are taking it two (or three for higher dosages) times a day. For smaller doses you may take it all at once. The following will help you find the dosage that is right for you:

Day 1:   1 capsule in the evening.
Day 2-3: 1 capsule in the morning or before lunch and 1 capsule in the evening.
Day 4-5: 1 capsule in the morning or before lunch and 2 capsules in the evening.

Day 6-7: 2 capsules in the morning or before lunch and 2 capsules in the evening.

Day 8-on: And so on.

Notes:

• If you get diarrhea and/or excessive watery elimination (sometimes common when determining your personal dosage the first few days), cut back the dosage so you have at least 2-3 firmer bowel movements a day. It is typical to have looser stools when cleansing.

• *If you don't see results from up to 6 capsules a day*, then keep slowly increasing the dosage evenly throughout the day (i.e. 3 capsules – 3 times a day, 4 capsules – 3 times a day and so on) until you finally start having at least 2-4 bowel movements a day. Then start reducing the amount of capsules taken, but make sure you are still having 2-4 bowel movements a day.

• For *best results* when cleansing, *follow Plan A or B in this book.*

How To Stay Healthy and In Shape

Most people will experience a thorough cleansing within 1-3 months, and achieve very noticeable weight loss and body shaping results. Everyone should do a 90 day program (at least) the first time they cleanse to help thoroughly cleanse and improve their digestive system, even though many will achieve their body shaping goals before that time. Also, it is helpful to do a thorough two-week cleansing once per calendar quarter.

Your "Secret Weapon" During Holidays & Vacations!

Sculpt n' Cleanse can also be used during times of heavy or "unhealthy" eating, like during holidays and vacations to help keep heavier meal's foods from stagnating in your system and contributing to constipation and weight gain.

#1 Rated Cleansing Supplement

Sculpt n' Cleanse **was recently rated the #1 cleansing supplement by** *Healthy Living Magazine*. **See the complete article at: www.reshapeforlife.com**

---

*These statements have not been evaluated by the Food and Drug Administration. This product is not intended to diagnose, treat, cure or prevent any disease.

AminoSculpt®

"The Original And Only Patented Collagen Formula"

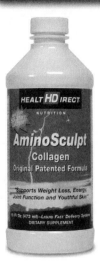

Collagen can help*:

- Reduce body fat
- Retain and promote muscle
- Firm and tone the body
- Support joint function
- Improve skin, hair and nail appearance
- Promote better sleep

Product Description

AminoSculpt is one of the best sources of protein available. Easily absorbable protein is extremely important during weight loss, loss, and anti-aging programs, as well as for older individuals.

As we age, the body's ability to digest protein becomes less efficient, and the body's ability to create and maintain collagen also diminishes. Since collagen is one of the most prevalent substances in the body, the effects from its loss are very visible. We get fine lines and wrinkles, our joints begin to stiffen and ache, our hair becomes lifeless and our body's muscle loses tone.

In order to counteract the loss of collagen, we can support our body's collagen by supplementing with a high-potency, bioavailable collagen, like *AminoSculpt*. No other supplement contains more collagen per tablespoon, or is more absorbable than *AminoSculpt*. Every tablespoon delivers eight grams of enzymatically predigested collagen that can be used by the body to firm and tone muscle, diminish the appearance of fine lines and wrinkles, add body to limp and lifeless hair, and increase joint function and flexibility. And if taken at bedtime when dieting, it can help to reduce body fat and inches.

Why *AminoSculpt* is different:

• **More Collagen:** *AminoSculpt* contains up to 284% more collagen than any other product available!

• **Collagen Protein:** *AminoSculpt*'s collagen protein is different from whey and all other proteins as it is the most natural and identical to the body; and it contains specific high nitrogen amino acids that the body lacks and needs as we age.

• **Best Absorption:** *AminoSculpt*'s proprietary natural predigested formula makes it the best absorbed and most bioavailable protein available.

• **Best Collagen:** *AminoSculpt* contains a proprietary and patented collagen formula, *COLLAPURE*™ (look for this name on the label to verify the authenticity). *AminoSculpt* is the only formula used by over 3,800 physicians and hospitals for over 32 years.

How to use *AminoSculpt*:

Take one tablespoon at bedtime with water (works best with 8 ounces) on an empty stomach (two, preferably 3 hours after eating). For increased results, take two tablespoons. If you eat late, still take *AminoSculpt*, as its patented natural enzyme hydrolysis method allows for complete and immediate absorption.

For Energy: AminoSculpt can be taken upon rising or any time during the day to support energy.

As a Protein Supplement or to Build Muscle: Take 1-2 tablespoons two - three times a day between meals. Or take it before and after your workout.

*These statements have not been evaluated by the Food and Drug Administration. This product is not intended to diagnose, treat, cure or prevent any disease.

Ready Fiber®
"The World's First Ready-To-Use, Liquid Fiber And Digestion Improving Supplement"

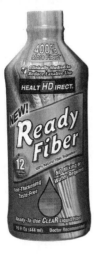

Fiber can help*:
- Support weight loss
- Improve regularity and digestive health
- Relieve bloating and upset stomachs
- Maintain healthy cholesterol within normal levels
- Maintain healthy blood sugar within normal levels

Product Description

Adequate fiber consumption has been shown to help increase weight loss, improve regularity, relieve occasional constipation, relieve bloating, reduce cholesterol, maintain healthy blood pressure, reduce blood sugar swings, and relieve digestive problems. Fiber affects weight loss by helping to: 1) reduce blood sugar absorption and insulin spikes; 2) slow the transit time of foods in the intestines, which promotes weight loss by decreasing the number of calories that are absorbed; and 3) increase a person's feeling of fullness.

Ready Fiber makes it easy to consume enough fiber as it contains a highly concentrated dose of fiber (12 grams) in a single taste-free ounce. *Ready Fiber* also contains FOS (fructo-oligosaccharides), a prebiotic, which helps improve digestive health and immune function. FOS stimulates and strengthens the growth and development of beneficial bacteria in your digestive system, which is important in controlling the overgrowth of yeasts such as Candida albicans. Studies have also shown that FOS can promote the absorption of calcium and magnesium (which makes it especially great for women).

Since 9 out of 10 Americans do <u>not</u> consumer the daily recommended amount of fiber (25 grams for women, 38 grams for men), it makes sense to supplement you diet.

Why *Ready Fiber* is different:

- **More Fiber:** *Ready Fiber contains nearly 400% more fiber than the leading supplements.* One ounce of *Ready Fiber* is equivalent to consuming *four*, 8-ounce glasses of gritty fiber powder, or *22* fiber capsules.

- **SAFE:** *Ready Fiber* does <u>NOT</u> affect the absorption of other supplements or medicines like other fiber supplements.

- **Prebiotic Support:** *Ready Fiber* contains the prebiotic FOS for additional support for digestive issues and cleansing programs.

- **Ready-To-Use & Versatile:** *Ready Fiber* can be used "as is" with NO water or mixing required, or can be mixed with any hot or cold food or beverage without changing either taste or texture.

How to Use *Ready Fiber*:

Take 2 teaspoons (10ml), two to four times per day as needed. *Ready Fiber* can be taken "as is" or added to ANY hot or cold food or beverage. Always consume adequate amounts of water throughout the day when taking any fiber product.

---

*These statements have not been evaluated by the Food and Drug Administration. This product is not intended to diagnose, treat, cure or prevent any disease.

Carb Cheater®

"Comprehensive Blood Sugar And Insulin Management Formula"

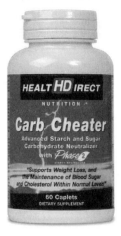

Carb Cheater can help*:

- Support weight loss programs
- Support blood sugar and insulin within normal levels
- Maintain cholesterol within normal levels
- Aid in lowering the glycemic index of foods

Product Description

C*arb Cheater* is an all-natural, carbohydrate neutralizing, weight management supplement. Many carbohydrates (starches and sugars) are considered "empty calories," since they are either burned off as energy or stored as fat. Excessive carbohydrate consumption can also overly increase levels of blood sugar and insulin, which can increase body fat (especially in the waistline); and cause bloating, sleepiness after meals, diabetic conditions and other health problems.

The ingredients in *Carb Cheater* are clinically studied to help reduce the absorption of starch carbohydrate calories and can help reduce some of the negative effects that simple carbohydrates have on blood sugar and insulin levels. *Carb Cheater* does not interfere with the absorption or body's utilization of any vitamins, minerals, proteins, fatty acids, or other nutrients.

Why *Carb Cheater* is different:

• **Four-in-One Supplement:** *Carb Cheater* contains 12 powerful weight loss, blood sugar and insulin supporting ingredients including: *Phase 2, Gymnema Sylvestre, Fenugreek Seed, Alpha Lipoic Acid, Green Tea Extract, Banaba Leaf Extract, Chromium Amino Acid Chelate, Vanadium, Panax Ginseng P.E., Bee Pollen Powder, Royal Jelly, and Eleuthero Root.*

• **Affects ALL Carbohydrates:** *Carb Cheater* helps reduce some of the negative effects of both starch and sugar carbohydrates.

• *Carb Cheater* contains **NO Stimulants!**

How to Use:

Take 1-2 caplets with water at the beginning of meals (preferably a few minutes before) containing carbohydrates. Three caplets can be taken with larger meals if desired. Be sure to drink at least 8-10 glasses of water a day when using *Carb Cheater*. *To help maintain your overall weight and overall health*: Take 1 or 2 caplets with your lunch and/or evening meals, or the meal containing the most carbohydrates. *Avoid* taking digestive enzymes containing "amylase," as this enzyme can offset some of the starch neutralizing effects of *Carb Cheater*.

When using *Carb Cheater* only 1-2 times per day, preferably use it:
1) During later meals such as lunch and especially dinner – as the meals containing carbohydrates later in the day are typically converted to fat, if they are not used as energy;
2) During your largest carbohydrate containing meal, especially those containing starch and sugar restricted foods, or alcohol.
3) Always with a "cheat" meal.

*These statements have not been evaluated by the Food and Drug Administration. This product is not intended to diagnose, treat, cure or prevent any disease.

Nature's Optimal Nutrition®

"The #1 Rated All-Purpose, Super-Energy, High-Potency, Anti-Aging Multivitamin With Over 220 Vital Nutrients"

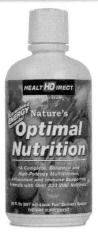

Nature's Optimal Nutrition can help*:

- Increase energy levels
- Support healthy immune function
- Support cardiovascular health
- Provide antioxidant protection
- Provide vital phytonutrients and nutrient co-factors not found in other multivitamin products

Product Description

Numerous published studies, including those from the United States Department of Agriculture (USDA), over the last 50 years have continuously shown evidence that our food's vitamin and mineral content continues to diminish. Commonly eaten vegetables have shown a vitamin and mineral content depletion of up to 60%, including vital nutrients like Vitamins C and B, potassium, magnesium and calcium. Also, many of us unknowingly deplete even more of the nutrients by the way we prepare our foods (cooking, heating, microwaving, etc).

Furthermore, the Daily Values (DV) set by the USDA were originally set as a minimum daily requirement for maintaining our health, and *not for ensuring optimal health*. And individuals who diet, exercise or are under stressful situations (life, family, work) often require additional nutrient support. Based on these facts, it makes sense to use a multivitamin/mineral supplement as a "nutritional insurance" policy.

Supplements

Nature's Optimal Nutrition is the most comprehensive, and cost-effective supplement available as it contains a complete, balanced and high-potency blend of over 220 immune and energy supporting vital nutrients – including 21 vitamins, 69 minerals, 6 super strength antioxidants, 30 herbal extracts, 35 fruit and vegetable extracts, 13 amino acids, plus much more! Plus, *Nature's Optimal Nutrition's* liquid delivery system provides immediate, easier and more efficient nutrient absorption than tablets, capsules and powders.

Why *Nature's Optimal Nutrition* is different:

- **Guaranteed Energy:** *Nature's Optimal Nutrition* provides you a guaranteed boost of energy you'll feel <u>without</u> any stimulants.

- **100% All-Natural, Vegetarian and Tastes Great!**

- **Cost-Effective and Convenient:** *Nature's Optimal Nutrition* replaces the need for taking 7-10 pills and buying 10 different supplements <u>with</u> <u>an</u> <u>average</u> <u>savings</u> <u>of</u> <u>over</u> $60 <u>per</u> <u>month</u>! Also, it does NOT require refrigeration.

How to use *Nature's Optimal Nutrition*:
Take 1 ounce (2 tablespoons) per day (children 6-11 can take half this dose). Take with meals (ideally with breakfast). *Nature's Optimal Nutrition* can be mixed with water or your favorite beverage. Refrigeration is unnecessary, unless you prefer it cold.
For Best Results: Take 1 additional serving during the day for the first 7 days. ***For Energy:*** An additional serving can be taken during the day (with 8-12 ounces of water). *Nature's Optimal Nutrition* is also an potent energy booster when taken prior to exercising. When using <u>later</u> <u>in</u> <u>the</u> <u>day</u>, you can take it on an empty stomach.

#1 Rated Multivitamin

Nature's Optimal Nutrition **was independently rated the #1 multivitamin of its kind. See the complete article at: www.reshapeforlife.com.**

---

*These statements have not been evaluated by the Food and Drug Administration. This product is not intended to diagnose, treat, cure or prevent any disease.

Optimal Omega HP®

"A High Potency, Super Antioxidant, Anti-Aging Omega-3 Fish Oil Supplement"

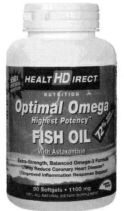

Omega-3 Fish Oils can help support*:

• Weight loss programs
• Healthy cholesterol within normal levels
• Healthy vision and eye health
• Joint mobility
• Improved inflammation response
• Improved memory and concentration
• Improved mood

Other Benefits:

Consumption of Omega-3 fatty acids may reduce the risk of coronary heart disease. The FDA evaluated this and found that although there is scientific evidence supporting this, the evidence is not conclusive.

Product Description

Since their discovery in the 1970's, <u>thousands</u> <u>of</u> <u>studies</u> have documented the health promoting and life-enhancing benefits of Omega-3 fatty acids (EPA and DHA). In fact, people in different parts of the world where high amounts of Omega-3's are consumed have shown the longest life-spans and some of the lowest death rates from diseases. Diets rich in Omega-3's can support healthy hearts, joints, immune systems, skin and nervous systems, mood, mental function and a healthy inflammation process.

Studies have also shown that Omega-3 fish oils, when combined with exercise, led to reduction in fat mass; while recent preliminary studies on both Omega 3's and *Astaxanthin* showed these nutrients could reduce body fat by boosting your body's fat metabolism. Also, new cutting-edge research shows that Omega-3 fish oil supplements improve insulin sensitivity.

Supplements

Optimal Omega HP is the world's first Omega-3 fish oil in a 100% natural, balanced one-to-one ratio of EPA and DHA, combined with the antioxidant, *Astaxanthin.*

Astaxanthin is an all-natural, ocean-derived powerful antioxidant clinically shown to protect the skin, eyes and body's tissues and cells from aging and damage, as well as from UV exposure from the sun. *Astaxanthin* is what gives salmon its pinkish-orange color and some additional health benefits not present in other fish oil Omega-3 products. Each *Optimal Omega HP* softgel contains as much *Astaxanthin* as found in a seven ounce serving of Wild Atlantic Salmon.

Why *Optimal Omega HP* is different:

- **Powerful Antioxidant:** Contains *Astaxanthin.* shown to be 550 times stronger than Vitamin E in antioxidant activity.

- **Cost-Effective/MORE Omega-3's:** Each softgel of *Optimal Omega HP* contains 72-100% MORE Omega-3's than the leading brands. You'd have to buy 2-3 bottles of other fish oil products to get the same amount of Omega-3's in one bottle of *Optimal Omega HP*, so it SAVES YOU MONEY!

- **Convenience:** *Optimal Omega HP* is super concentrated with more Omega-3's, so you'll need to take fewer softgels.

- **Best Quality:** Made from only deep, small, cold-water fish and manufactured in a pharmaceutically DRUG-LICENSED facility using a five-step, detoxification process with molecular distillation.

- **Contaminant-Free:** Third-party certified to be FREE of detectible levels of mercury, heavy metals, PCB's, pesticides, and over 240 other contaminants.

- **No Fishy Taste or Odor!**

How to use *Optimal Omega HP*:

Take 2-3 capsules per day, preferably with meals. For increased results, 4-6 capsules can be taken daily.

*These statements have not been evaluated by the Food and Drug Administration. This product is not intended to diagnose, treat, cure or prevent any disease.

Binge Buster®

"A Triple-Action Fat Burning And Appetite Control Spray"

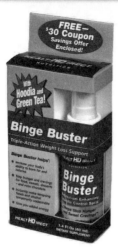

Binge Buster can help*:

- Support the burning of fat and calories
- Reduce binge eating
- Stop cravings for sweets, desserts, and even chocolate
- Make tempting foods taste undesirable

Product Description

Successful weight loss and weight management requires controlling the amount of food you eat. Because our bodies produce powerful and necessary impulses to eat, controlling our food consumption is often the most difficult part of dieting. *Binge Buster* helps work with your body's natural responses to stop hunger and sweet cravings and helps block the sweetness sensation and your appetite for sugar – even for chocolate!

Starting in your thirties, your body's metabolism can slow down, causing weight gain. To help maintain a healthy metabolism level, *Binge Buster* contains key nutrients like *Green Tea* to enhance your metabolism and your body's natural ability to burn fat and calories – without harmful stimulants.

Supplements

Why *Binge Buster* is different:

- **Immediate Results:** *Binge Buster*'s oral spray delivery system works quickly, unlike pill and capsule products.

- **Authentic Hoodia Gordonii (20:1 Extract):** *Binge Buster's* oral spray delivery system simulates the original <u>oral</u> use of Hoodia by the Kalahari Bushman by allowing an interaction of the ingredients with the tongue, saliva and buccal mucosa (which capsule and pill Hoodia products do not).

- **Four Other Synergistic Ingredients:** Also contains *Green Tea Extract, Peppermint Oil, Gymnema Sylvestre and Chromium.*

- Great chocolate-mint flavor.

How to Use:

Use one (1) or more sprays on the inside of the cheek, hold for 15-30 seconds and then swallow. For best results use at least two (2) sprays of *Binge Buster,* four (4) times a day (preferably before meals) – or whenever sudden craving for any foods, sweets or chocolate not in your eating plan arises.

---

*These statements have not been evaluated by the Food and Drug Administration. This product is not intended to diagnose, treat, cure or prevent any disease.

MSM®
"An Ultra-Purified Organic Sulfur Supplement"

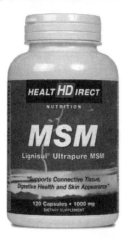

MSM can help support*:

- Healthy digestive function
- Joint function
- Healthy hair, skin and nails
- Energy levels

Product Description

MSM *(Methyl-Sulfonyl-Methane)* is a naturally occurring organic source of biologically available nutritional sulfur. *MSM* plays many important roles in the body including: maintaining the structure of the proteins; helping with the formation of keratin which is essential for hair and nail growth; aiding in the production of immunoglobulins, which maintains the immune system; and catalyzing the chemical reactions which change food into energy. Organic sulfur is also used by the body to create healthy cells and build strong connective tissue like cartilage, tendons, and ligaments.

   Sulfur-rich *MSM* is found in many fresh foods, but is easily destroyed by cooking and most food processing. Modern diets, as well as the natural aging process, result in *MSM* deficiencies in many people, making supplementation more important than ever. *MSM* and its related compounds are the source of 85 percent of the sulfur found in all living organisms. Many researchers believe that sulfur, an abundant element in the body, is a sorely neglected mineral nutrient and plays an indispensable role in human nutrition.

Supplements

This *MSM* is manufactured to the highest quality standards and third party tested to ensure a 99.9% purity level. It is an all-natural form of *MSM*. Cheaper *MSM* is not manufactured to the same quality standards, nor is it third party tested for purity.

Why this *MSM* is different:

- **Ultra Pure:** It is the first brand of *MSM* specifically developed as an "ultra-pure" nutritional supplement.

- **Third-Party Tested:** It is third-party tested to ensure a 99.9% purity level.

How to Use:

For a regular maintenance dose, take 2-4 capsules per day as needed. The *maximum amount* needed will vary among individuals. As a general rule, 1 capsule per 50 lbs. of body weight two times per day. For most women that would be 2-3 capsules twice a day; and most men, 3-4 twice a day. Start by taking one capsule, twice a day and increase by adding 2 capsules every day until the desired amount is reached (i.e., 1 and 1, 2 and 2, 3 and 3, etc). Stay at this level until desired results are achieved.

It is also wise to do a saturation dose of around 4000 mg (4 capsules) twice a day for at least a week when beginning *MSM*.

Notes: Divide your doses of *MSM* so you are taking it 10-12 hours apart. Users sometimes notice more energy, so take it during earlier meals if this affects you in the evenings. *MSM* can be taken on an empty stomach.

Premium Whey Protein Isolate™

"Pure, All-Natural Protein Supplement"

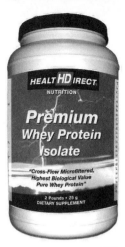

Supplemental Whey Protein can help*:

- Provide easily absorbable and digestible protein
- Ensure sufficient protein is consumed and utilized by the body during dieting
- Spare, maintain and build lean muscle tissue
- Support immune function

Product Description

After water and oxygen, protein is one of the most prevalent and essential nutrient and structural substances in our bodies. Our muscles, organs, glands, bones, teeth, skin, hair and nails are all made up of protein. It is a constituent of every cell, and the functional element in our hormones, enzymes and glandular secretions. Protein is also critical for tissue growth and repair.

When you do not have enough protein in your diet, your body will break down your muscle tissue to meet its protein needs. When this happens during dieting, you can end up with an un-toned body and loose skin. Also, *when you diet or exercise, your body requires more protein than normal.*

While food is the preferred source for protein, it cannot always be digested and assimilated well by the body. Aging, stress and digestive conditions can all contribute towards improperly digested and absorbed proteins and the resulting protein deficiency. This is why it makes sense to use protein supplements. *Premium*

Whey Protein Isolate is one of the purest supplemental food sources of all-natural, easily absorbable, and bioavailable protein.

Why this *Premium Whey Protein Isolate* is different:

• **All Natural**
• **Highest Biological Value**
• **Cross-Flow Microfiltered**
• **No Artificial Sweeteners** - NO Aspartame, Sucralose, or Acesulfame-K
• **No Refined Sugars, Sucrose, or Maltodextrin**
• **Rich In Anti-Catabolic Branch Chain Amino Acids (BCAAs)** – aids in preventing lean muscle tissue breakdown
• **Rich In B-lactoglobulin, A-Lactalbumin, Immunogoblins and Glycomacro Peptides**
• **High Protein Content:** 25 grams per serving
• **Low Carb:** 3.5 grams per serving
• **Low Fat:** less than 1 gram per serving
• **No Gluten, Corn, Egg, or Preservatives**
• **Low In Lactose**
• **Easily Digested And Bioavailable To The Body**
• **Mixes Instantly And Easily**
• **Delicious, Rich Chocolate Flavor**

How to Use *Premium Whey Protein Isolate*:

Mix one (1) scoop (25 grams of protein) with your favorite beverage like water, milk, or juice. You can even mix it into your favorite foods, like oatmeal, yogurt, etc. Athletes and those on heavy weight training or bodybuilding routines may consume even more (40-50 grams). Also *Premium Whey Protein Isolate* is the best protein supplement to use in a *post-workout shake* as it is quickly absorbed and utilized by the body.

---

*These statements have not been evaluated by the Food and Drug Administration. This product is not intended to diagnose, treat, cure or prevent any disease.

Exercise

Always consult a physician before starting any exercise program.

"Firming, Toning, RESHAPING Your Body - And Boosting Your Metabolism"

Let's start by my saying that *I strongly recommend you exercise* - if not for this program - for your overall health and well-being.

For maximum body reshaping, like you see in the before and after photos of myself and my clients throughout this book, you need to exercise. No "magic wonder pill" will ever shape and firm your body like exercise.

Three of the best reasons you should exercise are:

1. *Exercise preserves and builds muscle* - firming, toning and shaping your body – which will help you look and feel younger.

2. Exercise helps *increase your metabolism,* whereas low-calorie diet programs without exercise usually show a 20% drop in a dieter's metabolism. In fact, certain types of exercise can help your metabolism stay elevated up to 48 hours afterwards!

3. Also, I have found it is much *easier to stay on an eating regimen* or *diet when exercise is included.* The two create positive cycles that support one another. Your body shaping results will come much quicker, which motivates you to stay on your diet, which in turn motivates you to exercise.

And I Don't Have To Live In The Gym?

People often have the wrong impression that they have to spend a lot of time exercising - this is wrong. Most are usually shocked when they learn that I only exercised 30 minutes to 1 hour maximum (with weights) – and only 3 times a week! That's all!

As I started this program, a friend of mine, Dr. Vicky Vodon, encouraged me to run. I hate running and argued, "Name one animal that runs 6 miles a day to stay in shape" (I heard a doctor say this

Exercise

once, and it sounded like a great comeback to use).

Well, my argument didn't hold up well with her, so I gave running (more like slow jogging) a shot. In only a very brief period, I started losing too much weight, too quickly (tough problem to have for a guy who had trouble losing weight before)! Because of this, I stopped and just did weights 3 times a week.

I am not saying to skip aerobic activities, like running - I encourage it - especially if you like it or are already doing it. It was just too much exercise for me then. Nowadays, I highly recommend speed walking (walking at a faster, controlled pace). It is easier on the body and more enjoyable for most people.

The point of all this is that *you should exercise*, but you really do not need as much exercise as most people think.

IMPORTANT
"If You Can't Or Don't Exercise, Then Read This..."

If you cannot exercise or do not for any reason, then I STRONGLY RECOMMEND YOU:

Take *AminoSculpt* (preferably twice a day – once at bedtime and once immediately upon rising).

Aside from exercise, the only other way to preserve muscle is to consume and *absorb* sufficient amounts of protein. *AminoSculpt* (collagen protein) is the most bioavailable and best protein for preserving, building and maintaining lean muscle (especially if you don't exercise). *AminoSculpt* also contains specific amino acids that have been shown to help optimize Growth Hormone levels in the body. This can also help build muscle.

Also, because a lot of people do not fully absorb protein foods (because of aging, illnesses, stress, or digestive issues), quality supplements like *AminoSculpt* and also adding a quality *protein shake (meal replacement)* can really assist them. Both are easier to digest so you absorb more protein than food.

Recommended Exercise

OK, you have been checked out by a physician and have been given the A-ok to exercise (and I recommend you show any routines or ways of exercising mentioned in this book or any other source to your physician before starting).

If you are an experienced exerciser or have routines that work well for you, you are welcome to follow them - just incorporate some of the guidelines and tips that I cover. This section will provide you with some new ideas and insights, so please review it.

Something For Everyone - Take Your Pick...

If you are not currently exercising, I cannot emphasize enough that <u>any type of physical activity</u> is better than nothing. I'll cover different types of exercise available to you. Also, many people always ask me what I did – so I've included my weight training routine (which I have adapted for women and beginners).

There are <u>three basic kinds of exercise</u>. Understanding the differences will help you achieve a balanced body. They each contribute to total fitness so it's important to work to eventually include them all in your life. They are:

1. <u>Aerobic Exercise</u>: This increases the amount of oxygen delivered to your muscles to allow them to work <u>longer</u>. This includes all the exercises listed below *other than* weight and resistance band training, pilates, and some forms of yoga.

2. <u>Resistance Exercise</u>: This <u>strengthens</u> <u>and</u> <u>builds</u> muscles to work harder and longer before becoming exhausted. This includes weight and resistance band training, and pilates.

3. <u>Flexibility Exercise</u>: This <u>lengthens</u> the muscles to counteract the shortening that can happen through age, inactivity, and other fitness activities. Stretching forms of exercise also include yoga and pilates. Also work towards including non-exercise stretching with other forms of exercise as it is great for improving muscle tone, shape, and can help alleviate structural aches and pains. For this kind of stretching, I recommend the book "*Stretching*" by Bob Andersen or, even better, "*Eat, Move and Be Healthy*" by Paul Chek.

The following is a list that includes common types of exercise that can be used.

- Weight training
- Resistance band training
- Jogging, running, sprinting
- Aerobics
- Trampoline bouncing*
- Stair-walking
- Walking

- Pilates
- Yoga
- Spinning
- Bicycling
- Swimming
- Kick boxing
- Dancing (fast paced)

__Note:__ We have all seen these little round trampolines in our neighbor's garage, typically unused with rust on them. I highly recommend them, as they are one of the best sources of aerobic exercise. It is easy on the joints; has numerous benefits for the immune system; is convenient for your home; and is great for rainy or snowy days, or during hot humid weather when you do not want to be outside.

My friend, Kirsten (you saw pictures in the first section), used the mini-trampoline 3-4 times a week for 20-45 minutes each time. She also did her weight training 2-3 times a week to get all her results in 27 days - and she had not done any exercise for four years prior to this!

"Inch By Inch, Exercise Is A Cinch!"

If exercise is a big deal to you, do something like walking a block or two. Every day add an extra block to your route. Then after you are walking a further distance (45-60 minutes) – pick up the pace to a light, very slow jog.

Don't compare yourself to others – just do what you can – add to it – and **be proud that you did it**. Before long, you will surprise yourself. Do not overdo it, and remember, *"Inch by inch, exercise is a cinch. Yard by yard, it tends to be hard."* Just a little more each time will bring results.

Everyday physical activities can also help improve your shape and health, so include them as much as you can. Some examples are:

- Washing windows and floors (45-60 minutes)
- Gardening (45 minutes)
- Walking instead of driving
- Washing and waxing a car (45-60 minutes)
- Raking leaves (30 minutes)
- Taking the stairs instead of an elevator

My Personal Recommendation...

The best form of exercise on a weight loss program is *resistance training*. As covered before, this is the best way to preserve lean muscle, increase your metabolism, shape your body, and burn fat!

Why Resistance Training Is Superior – The EXTRA BENEFITS...

Resistance training is superior to other forms of exercise as it *preserves, builds, and strengthens muscle*; can strengthen *and* improve joints; can increase bone density (only resistance exercise does this); burns more calories than other exercise *afterwards* (when not exercising); and can stimulate the release of Growth Hormone naturally.

Growth Hormone increases your metabolism, mobilizes your fat stores, and helps build and repair muscle. It is your "youth hormone." Your body naturally secretes more of it when you are younger - which is one reason why you can eat more and stay lean - and why you build muscle and recover from injuries quicker. When you are older, you still have plenty of Growth Hormone, but not as much is released like when you were younger. The best way to naturally increase the release of Growth Hormone is resistance (weight) training.

Ideally, for optimal weight loss and overall health, I recommend:

1. *Resistance Training* three times a week (for 30 minutes to 1 hour maximum), and if you can, include some...

Exercise

2. ***Low-Intensity Aerobic Exercise*** two to three days a week (for 20 minutes to 1 hour). As discussed earlier, aerobic types of exercise include: jogging, running, walking, biking, treadmills, stair masters, trampoline bouncing, etc.

> *Note:* The best exercise you can do is *resistance training*, and preferably with weights. If you only do one of the above – pick resistance training for 3 days a week – the results will amaze you!

These are two samples of what your weekly schedule can look like:

Sunday	Monday	Tuesday	Wednesday	Thursday	Friday	Saturday
Off	Weights	Off	Weights	Off	Weights	Off

OR

If you include aerobic exercise 2-3 times a week your schedule can look like this:

Sunday	Monday	Tuesday	Wednesday	Thursday	Friday	Saturday
Off	Weights	Aerobic	Weights	Aerobic	Weights	Aerobic

Ideally, resistance training should be in the morning as that is the best time to affect the release of Growth Hormone. Including aerobic training will help you lose weight faster. But, if you leave any days out - leave an aerobic day out, not a resistance training day.

Note: If you do them both in the same workout, always do resistance training first, and then do aerobic exercise.

Don't burn yourself out by being overly anxious to do a lot. The first weekly schedule is sufficient for most, as it provides proper rest and recuperation for your muscles and your nervous system.

> ### The Bottom Line For Getting Results With Exercise Is:
>
> ***It's not how much you work out – it's the quality.***
>
> To focus on quality: 1) Use good exercise form, and 2) push yourself continuously (slowly at first if you're a beginner).

"You Can't Hide Fat With A Back Picture"

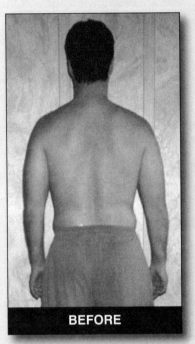
BEFORE

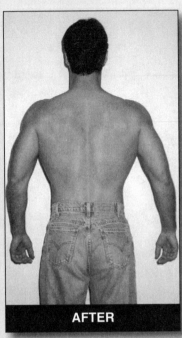
AFTER

I prefer back photos when showing before and after pictures, because <u>back</u>-<u>fat</u> <u>can't</u> <u>be</u> <u>hidden</u>!

Notice: My lower back-fat (love handles) are gone; my soft, narrow shoulders are now lean and shapely. You can see muscle development and shape in the upper back. The back also has a nice V-shape running down to the waistline. The back of the arms (triceps) also have shape and improved muscle tone, and I have lost the fat (this is a common problem area for women). And, my hips have lost the fatty width and are now shapely and toned.

This is why you want to preserve and gain muscle when dieting as you will look younger and shapelier. *A note for women:* Genetically, men will tend to shape into a <u>stronger</u>, <u>more</u> <u>muscular</u> <u>look</u>. <u>Women's</u> <u>bodies</u> <u>will</u> <u>develop</u> <u>into</u> <u>a</u> <u>firmer</u>, <u>toned</u>, <u>shapelier</u>, <u>and</u> <u>feminine</u> <u>look</u>, even if weights are used.

Exercise

Exercise Routines

The following routines will reshape, tone and build your body. They are structured to increase your body's natural Growth Hormone production, stimulate fat loss, and build lean muscle tissue. Here is a routine you can use that will produce fast results.

Fat-Burning Resistance Training Plan

These routines provide a complete body workout. They are strategically designed to target all the muscles of the body at different angles. This provides maximum muscle shape and physique development. The exercises also indirectly stimulate some of the same muscles in the different workouts, so you do not have to exercise a body part more than once a week. These workouts are excellent for beginners, and done more intensely, will even sufficiently challenge intermediate and advanced lifters.

Helpful Workout Definitions

To make sure you get off to a good start with your workouts, here are some helpful definitions for the terms used below in the workouts and in this section.

- **Reps (repetitions):** The number of times you continuously perform that exercise.

- **Sets:** When you do a number of repetitions (reps) continuously, that is one "set".

- **Rest:** The time you will rest between each set.

- **Intensity:** This is the amount of work or "stress" (a good thing in this case) you place on the muscles exercised. Intensity is determined by: 1) the length of time (rest) between sets; 2) the weight (resistance) used; 3) continually increasing the weight used (discussed in upcoming "*Workout Notes and Reminders*"); and

4) your "form" or doing the exercise correctly.

Note: Descriptions on how to do these exercises can be found on the pages 113-136 in this section entitled *"Exercise Descriptions and Instructions"*.

Workout 1: Chest, Arms, Lower Abs (Monday)			Sets*	Reps	Rest
Bodypart		Exercise	Sets*	Reps	Rest
Chest	1	Bench Press*	2	10-12	90 sec
	2	Flat-Bench Flyes	1	10-12	90 sec
Biceps	3a	Barbell or Dumbbell Curl*	2	10-12	60 sec
Triceps	3b	Push Downs with Bar	2	10-12	60 sec
Biceps	4a	Incline Bench Dumbbell Curls	2	10-12	60 sec
Triceps	4b	Standing Bar Extensions	2	10-12	60 sec
Abs	5a	Reverse Crunches	2	12-15	60 sec
	5b	Cross Crunches	2	12-15	60 sec
Workout 2: Legs, Upper Abs (Wednesday)					
Quadriceps, Hamstrings, Glutes	1	Squats* or Step Ups*	2	10-12	90 sec
	2	Lunges	2	10-12	90 sec
	3a	Leg Extensions	2	10-12	90 sec
	3b	Leg Curls*	2	10-12	90 sec
Calves	4	Standing Calf Raises*	2	12-15	60 sec
	5	Seated Calf Raises	2	12-15	60 sec
Abs	6	Crunches	2	12-15	60 sec
Workout 3: Back, Shoulders, Lower Abs (Friday)					
Back	1a	Machine Pull Down or Pull Up*	2	10-12	60 sec
Shoulders	1b	Machine (or Barbell) Press*	2	10-12	60 sec
Back	2a	One Arm Dumbbell Rows	2	10-12	60 sec
Shoulders	2b	Side Lateral Raises	2	10-12	60 sec
Back	3	Straight Arm Pull Downs	2	12-15	60 sec
Abs	4	Reverse Crunches	2	12-15	60 sec
	5	Cross Crunches	2	12-15	60 sec

* On these exercises, do an additional 1-2 light warm-up sets of 12-15 repetitions with 50% of weight you will work out with prior to and in addition to the above.

Learning and *perfecting* the above exercises will give you the *foundational knowledge* to later expand and easily learn other exercises.

Exercise

Using exotic equipment (like kettle balls, bosu balls, etc.) *as a beginner* is unnecessary, and from my experience, unwise. Mastering the basics will allow you to get the full benefit from these other devices later on, as well as avoid injury while you're beginning.

Home or Travel Exercise Routine

The following routine is designed for those who need to exercise from home, occasionally can't make the gym, and /or travel.

The routine incorporates many of the same exercises, but uses either dumbbells and/or resistance bands (convenient if you're traveling). Descriptions of these exercises can be found at the end of the upcoming *Exercise Descriptions and Instructions* section. The *Workout Notes and Reminders* still apply.

Bodypart	Exercise	Sets	Reps	Rest
Legs	Lunges	2	12-15	60 sec
Chest	Push Ups	2	15-20	60 sec
Back	One Arm Dumbbell Rows	2	12-15	60 sec
Shoulders	Dumbbell Press	2	12-15	60 sec
Biceps	Dumbbell Curls	2	12-15	60 sec
Triceps	Dumbbell Kickbacks or Band Extensions	2	12-15	60 sec
Calves	One Leg Standing Calf Raises	2	15-20	30 sec
Abs	Crunches or Cross Crunches	2	12-15	60 sec

Notes:
- Do this routine every other day, three times per week.
- Increase the repetitions (13-15, 18-20, 20-25) occasionally for variation.
- Continually increase your weights (or band strength). You can also add one more set for each exercise when you can increase the workload and intensity.
- For a variation, you can do the exercises in a "circuit." A circuit is when you do one of each exercise, continuously going to the next exercise without resting, then resting 60-120 seconds after you have finished one rotation of all the exercises. Then do it again, so when finished, you have completed two sets of each exercise.

Workout Notes and Reminders

- Monday/Wednesday/Friday's are listed as a sample. You can adjust these days to fit your schedule (i.e. Tuesday/Thursday/ Saturday), but always keep one day off *in between* workouts.

- *A & B Exercises:* Exercises grouped under the same number (e.g., 1a and 1b) are to be *alternated*. For example, after doing a set of 1a, rest 60 seconds and then do a set of exercise 1b. After resting 60 seconds, return to set 1a, and so on (until all the sets of these exercises are completed). All other exercises (1, 2, 3, etc.) should be done in the order listed with the rest period indicated (60 or 90 sec).

- If you want to put more emphasis on working your legs, then do Workout 2 again after Workout 3 (before starting Workout 1 again). For example, Workout 1 (Mon), Workout 2 (Wed), Workout 3 (Fri), Workout 2 (the following Monday). Then start Workout 1 again on Wednesday and repeat this cycle.

- Do some light aerobic work for about 5-10 minutes before starting (stationary biking, etc.) to warm up your body.

- The speed at which a repetition is done should be 3-0-2 on all exercises - meaning *3 seconds* lowering the weight from the starting position, *0 seconds* at the bottom or middle of the exercise, and *2 seconds* lifting the weight back to the starting position. Do not pause at any place *during* the repetition.

- 60 or 90 seconds rest between all sets as indicated in the chart.

- Continuously increase the intensity. Use a weight you can do both "sets" with. When you achieve both sets with that weight for the full number of repetitions, increase the weight. For example, if you Bench Press 100 lbs., do it until you can do 2 sets of 12 for 100 lbs., then increase the weight to 110 (about 10%). Stay at this weight until you can do 2 sets of 12 with 110, then increase again. Always try to keep increasing the weight, but never sacrifice your "form" (correctly doing the exercise).

- Do not exercise longer than 1 hour. After your warm-up is

Exercise

completed, the routine is designed to last 30-50 minutes (including all rest periods).

- For maximum fat loss, *exercise first thing in the morning on an empty stomach.* Research shows this can increase fat loss by up to 300%! Drinking water and/or taking a tablespoon or two of *AminoSculpt* is encouraged. These are still considered an empty stomach.

- Drink plenty of water before and during exercise. Do not have sports drinks, as they are heavy in sugar and carbohydrates. Also, limit carbohydrate consumption before or during exercise. Your body will use them as fuel instead of utilizing your body fat.

- If you have been working out consistently (and intensely), take a week off every 4-5 weeks and then start back up. You can do light aerobic work during the week off if you prefer.

- Women can change the reps by adding 2-3 reps per set (i.e. instead of 10-12, do 12-15).

- Change the number of repetitions every 4 weeks, (Men: change the repetitions from 10-12 to 7-9, and women from 12-15 to 10-12), then 4 weeks later change back. You can also slightly alter some exercises every few weeks (by using dumbbells instead of barbells). These changes employ "muscle confusion," which further develops the muscle.

- Have a post-workout meal (shake) immediately following (within 1 hour) of intense exercise (see *"Don't Miss Your Critical Hour"* following this section).

- Avoid or strictly limit alcohol. Alcohol inhibits enzymes involved in energy production, hampers recovery, and decreases your natural production of testosterone (another anti-aging "youth hormone" that affects muscle growth, a better mood, and a feeling of well-being).

- Budget permitting, use a personal trainer. They can really accelerate your learning curve, help you get more out of exercise, and keep you disciplined.

Don't Miss Your "Critical Hour"

The *Critical Hour* is the hour immediately <u>after</u> *intense* <u>exercise</u>. During this hour it is estimated that your body can utilize up to 80% of the nutrients needed for recovery for the next 24 hours.

Exercise (intense, not passive) creates nutritional deficits that <u>need</u> <u>to</u> <u>be</u> <u>replaced</u>. If these go unattended, you will not recover properly and can possibly <u>lose</u> <u>muscle</u> instead of building it.

Your body prefers using carbohydrates as fuel. It stores these carbohydrates in the liver and muscle cells - these are known as glycogen. Glycogen gives you energy on demand!

The key to recovery is *getting the body's glycogen levels back to normal* – and you do this by ingesting carbohydrates (this is the one time when dieting it is OK to do this). Unlike other times of the day, carbohydrates - even in higher amounts – are typically <u>not</u> <u>stored</u> <u>as</u> <u>fat</u> when ingested at this time. They replenish glycogen.

Also, exercise lowers insulin levels, which is good for fat burning. But after exercise, you want to "spike" or raise your insulin levels, because <u>insulin</u> <u>will</u> <u>carry</u> <u>glucose</u> <u>and</u> <u>amino</u> <u>acids</u> <u>into</u> <u>the</u> <u>muscle</u> <u>cells</u> – which is important to muscle recovery, maintenance, and for those training to add muscle mass. This is why you need to <u>consume</u> <u>an</u> <u>easily</u> <u>digestive</u> <u>protein</u> <u>with</u> <u>carbohydrates</u> (preferably high glycemic ones – which is OK to do at this time only) to aid in the release of insulin to help get protein and nutrients to the muscles!

The **best post-workout meal** is a <u>liquid</u> <u>meal</u> <u>or</u> <u>shake</u> containing a <u>predigested</u> or easily absorbable protein powder supplement (25-40 grams), like whey protein isolate or concentrate, and carbohydrates (both complex and simple – higher glycemic). During the weight loss program in this book, 30-50 grams of carbohydrates should be the amounts used.

In the *Eating Plan Section* under *Post Exercise Protein Meal-Replacement Drinks*, I list some recipes for these. Consuming <u>a</u> <u>food</u> <u>meal</u> <u>after</u> <u>exercise</u> <u>is</u> <u>not</u> <u>as</u> <u>good</u> because of the time it takes to digest and absorb, but it is better than nothing.

Exercise

How you perform an exercise (previously referred to as "form") can make a big difference in *how quickly* you transform your body and *how good* it will look.

On the following pages that conclude this section, called *Exercise Descriptions and Instructions*, you will find very detailed descriptions with pictures on how to perform the exercises recommended in this book. Also included are special tips to ensure you get the most out of each exercise, as well as "*Do Not's*" which are common mistakes most people make when doing these exercises.

This information will dramatically shorten your learning curve – and will help you achieve a well-balanced and developed body much faster than most programs. If you are a beginner (or even an intermediate) here is the best and quickest way I have used to learn exercises over the past 25 years. Use these steps:

1. Before each workout (the night before up to before exercising): *Read* the instructions for the exercise you will be doing, and *picture in your mind* you doing them and the muscles used (this last part will be easier once you have done the exercises a few times).

2. During the workout: *Take this book with you to the gym* and read about each exercise before you do each set (brush up on what you are about to do).

Also, while doing the exercise *notice and feel the muscles you are working,* so you can learn how each exercise affects them (this helps to establish your mind-body connection).

3. After the workout (anytime, even later before bed): Re-read the instructions for the exercises you did that day. It always surprised me when I noticed a simple thing or tip I wasn't doing (even after doing this many times) that would make a big difference.

Before long, you won't need to follow the instructions, they will become part of your everyday skill set and knowing. Also, occasionally re-read them, as you will get different insights on doing the exercise, as your experience and body strength progresses.

One last reminder of an important step: DON'T BE SHY – take this book with you to the gym and reference it while doing the exercise. Those of us who are experienced have all done this too. Consider this book your own personal trainer!

The following exercise descriptions will teach you good *form* – but doing them is up to you! Unlike many authors, I have actually done these exercises (and routines). You'll notice this in the detail.

Workout 1: Chest, Arms, Abdominals

Bench Press (Chest)
- Lying face up on a bench; keep your back flat (with a slight arch in lower back), and your feet flat on the floor.
- Hold the bar with an overhead grip (palms facing away) with your hands slightly wider than your shoulders.
- Line up your elbows *under* the bar throughout the movement.
- Hold the bar above your chest, and then lower it smoothly to your mid-chest (nipples or right above), then *immediately* (without pausing) raise the bar back up in a straight line.
- **Tip:** Pinch your shoulder blades together slightly, have your shoulders down, and your chest up throughout the movement.
- Inhale as you lower the bar; exhale as you push the bar up.
- Have a "spotter" (another person) standing behind you (where your head is) to help you lift the bar off the rack and back.

The "Do Nots"
- Sink your chest or raise your shoulders off the bench.
- Overly arch your back, by pushing your feet too hard on the ground.
- Lower the bar towards your abdomen.
- Bounce the bar off your chest.

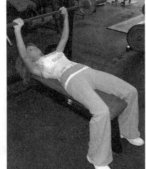
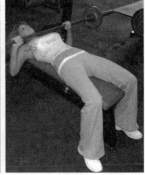

Exercise

Flat Bench Flyes (Chest)

- Lying face up on a bench, keep your back flat (<u>slight</u> arch in lower back), and feet flat on the floor.
- The palms of your hands face each other at top and throughout the movement and your *biceps* *always* face the ceiling through out the movement.
- Starting with your arms up and the dumbbells above your chest (4-6 inches apart), slowly lower the dumbbells until your arms reach shoulder level, or slightly below (you'll feel the stretch in your chest), then raise your arms back up, contracting your chest muscles at the top of the movement.
- Keep arms <u>slightly</u> <u>bent</u> <u>at</u> <u>the</u> <u>elbows</u> <u>at</u> <u>all</u> <u>times</u> - *especially at the bottom of the movement. Note: Your arms should be like you are hugging a tree through out the entire movement.*
- **Tip:** Pinch your shoulder blades together slightly, and keep your shoulders down and chest up throughout the movement.
- Inhale on your way down; exhale when you bring your arms back up.

The "Do Nots"
- Touch the dumbbells at the top.
- Sink (concave) your chest, or raise your shoulders off the bench.
- Bring your elbows towards your sides.
- Straighten your arms, or lock your elbows out.
- Rotate your palms downward.

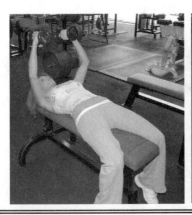 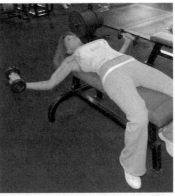

Barbell or Dumbbell Curls (Arms: Biceps)

- Stand with your feet shoulder width apart.
- Grip the bar shoulder width apart with your palms facing up.
- Curl bar from your thighs (starting point) to just shy of the chest (top of the movement) by a few inches and contract your biceps. Lower the bar back down *slowly*.
- Keep elbows in place, next to your sides at all times.
- **Tip:** Keep your wrists straight at all times. Focus on raising the pinky side of your hand towards the ceiling as you curl.
- Exhale as you lift the bar; inhale as you lower the bar.

The "Do Nots"

- Bend your body or swing the bar up from your waist.
- Bring your elbows up and/or forward, or away from your sides during the exercise.
- Relax your wrist, making it limp during the movement.
- Raise your heels or move your feet during the exercise.

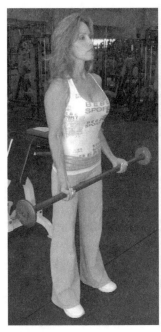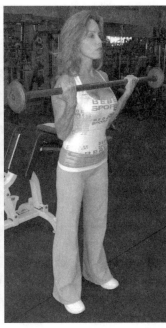

Exercise

Incline Bench Dumbbell Curls (Arms: Triceps)

- Set the bench at a 45 degree angle.
- Lie on the bench with your feet flat on floor.
- With your palms holding the dumbbells facing towards the front of your body (upwards), your arms will start straight down behind your torso. Curl the dumbbells up and contract your biceps at the top. Slowly lower them down (feeling the stretch in your biceps at the bottom).
- Keep your head on the bench or slightly elevated looking forward.
- Keep your elbows close to your sides.
- Get a complete stretch at the bottom of the movement.
- Exhale when lifting up; inhale when lowering the weights.

The "Do Nots"
- Swing your arms forward.
- Bring your elbows up and/or forward.
- Let your wrists be limp.
- Arch your back off of the bench.

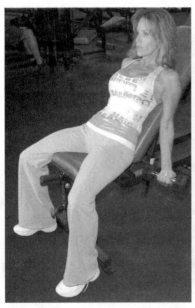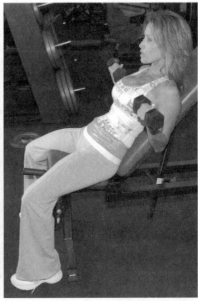

Triceps Cable Push-Downs (Arms: Triceps)

- Stand with your feet shoulder width apart.
- Grip the bar with your hads at a shoulder width apart or a little closer in.
- Keep the palms of your hands facing down over the bar.
- With the bar starting by your chest, push it straight down completely locking out your elbows. Straighten your arms at bottom of movement (so the bar is by your thighs).
- Keep your elbows <u>stationary</u> by your sides the entire time. Then slowly let the bar rise back up, controlling it.
- Exhale when pushing down; inhale when the weight comes back up.

The "Do Nots"
- Slide or rotate your hands on the bar during the movement
- Move your elbows forward, backwards, or outwards.
- Lift your feet off the ground.
- Bring the bar up over your chest (heart) level.
- Reach down (extending your shoulders) at the bottom of the movement.

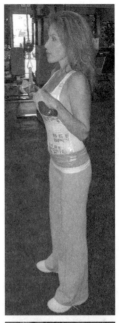

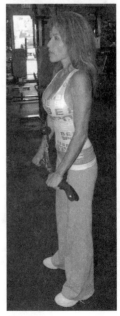

Exercise

Standing Cable-Triceps Extensions (Arms: Triceps)

- Grab the bar, bring it *overhead* and stand with your back to the machine.
- Stand with one foot slightly in front of the other.
- Slightly bend over at the waist (about 10-15 degrees).
- Grip the bar shoulder width or a little closer in.
- Start with the bar over your head (slightly behind your head), and lower the bar behind your head, then immediately press the bar back up until your arms lock at the elbow, and contract your triceps.
- Keep your elbows stationary.
- Keep the bar close to the top of your head during the exercise.
- Inhale when lowering the bar; exhale when pushing it back up.

The "Do Nots"
- Lift your feet off the floor at anytime during the exercise.
- Rotate your grip on the bar during the exercise.
- Keep the bar too far above your head.
- Let your elbows rotate outwards.

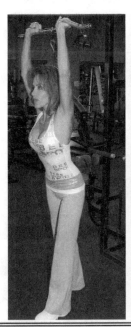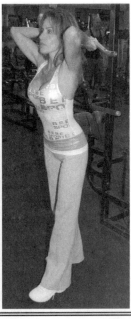

Reverse Crunches (Abdominals)

- Lying flat on a bench, bend your legs so your feet are on the bench.
- Grip the bench with both hands next to your ears.
- Keep your elbows about shoulder width apart.
- Contract your abs so as to bring your knees towards your elbows.
- This should *round-out* your back forcing the abs to contract.
- Keep a good solid grip and *pull slightly with your arms* as you perform each rep.
- Bring your feet back to the bench and repeat reps.
- Always keep your abs contracted throughout the entire movement. Do not relax them during reps.
- Exhale as your bring your legs up; inhale as you lower them.

The "Do Nots"
- Relax your abs <u>at</u> <u>any</u> <u>time</u>.
- Straighten your spine as you perform your reps.
- Hold your breath during the exercise.

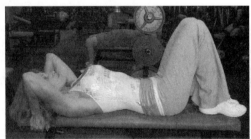

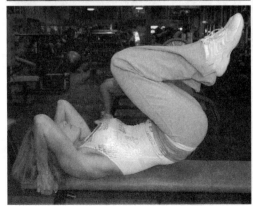

Exercise

Cross Crunches (Abdominals)

- Lie flat on your back on the floor with your legs bent and your feet flat on the floor.
- Hands *at the sides* of your head resting <u>gently</u> behind your ears (not locked together).
- Perform the abdominal crunch by bringing your right elbow towards your left knee and lifting your torso up as far as you can, and then return back down so your back is completely flat. Then bring your left elbow towards your right knee. (This is one rep).
- Your eyes should be looking at the ceiling the entire time.
- Your abs should contract and *keep your lower back flat against the floor at all times*.
- **Tip:** When crunching up, your neck, shoulders, head and arms should move <u>as one unit</u>. To avoid overextending or flexing your neck, pretend there is a small ball under your chin.
- Exhale as you crunch up; inhale as you lower your torso back down.

The "Do Nots"
- Never pull on the back of your head during the exercise.
- Jerk forward to perform a rep.
- Lift your feet off the floor during the exercise.
- Hold your breath during the exercise.
- Arch your lower back.

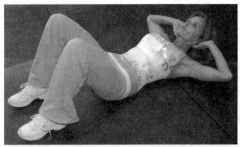

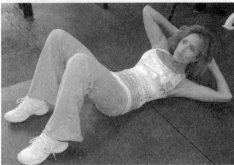

Squats (Legs: Quadriceps, Hamstrings, Glutes)

- Standing with feet shoulder width apart or slightly wider, angle your toes slightly outwards.
- Grip the bar with your hands a little wider than shoulder width.
- Place the bar behind your neck, across your shoulders and resting on your upper traps.
- Distribute your weight equally between your feet.
- Slowly bend your knees and hips, so you lower your body like you were sitting in a chair. Your knees will come forward slightly (and do not allow them to go past your toes), your butt will move back and down, and your torso will come forward slightly.
- The bottom of the position is when your thighs are *parallel* to the floor.
- Then start to raise the weight upwards (and focus on pushing your heels through the floor) and come under the weight.
- Always keep your back straight with chest out and keep your abdominals (abs) "tight" (contracted) the entire time.
- Your head should be straight and your eyes looking straight ahead.
- Inhale on the way down; forcefully exhale on the way up.

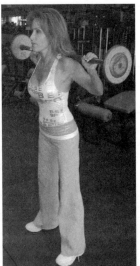
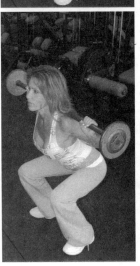

The "Do Nots"
- Lean over at the waist (or round out your back) when descending into your rep.
- Stand on your toes during the rep.

Exercise

- Allow your knees to wobble side to side or inward as you perform your reps.
- Put your head and neck back and look at the ceiling.

Step Ups – Dumbbell (Legs: Quadriceps, Hamstrings, Glutes)

- Face a box (bench or stairs).
- Step forward with one leg on top of box. Shift your body weight to the lead leg, (pressing through your heel) and move your body (and other leg) to a standing position on the box.
- Then, slowly step back off the box with your trailing leg and return to the starting position.
- Do not allow your body to overly lean forward while stepping up. You may slightly lean forward when you first go forward to start the movement up, but keep your back straight.
- Repeat process with the other leg. This completes one repetition (stepping up with each leg).
- **Tips:** Keep your abs tight while performing the exercise. Look forward at all times. Press weight through your heel. Contract (tighten) your hips and butt at the top of the movement.

The "Do Not's"
- Lean over at waist or round your back when stepping up.
- Put the weight on the toes of your lead foot when stepping up.
- Look down.

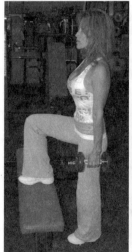
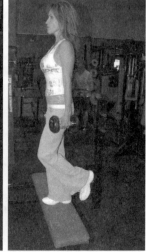

Lunges (Legs: Quadriceps, Hamstrings, Glutes)

- Stand with feet close together.
- Hold dumbbells in each hand.
- Keeping your torso erect, take a big step forward and descend slowly with your front leg forming a 90-degree angle at the knee joint and with your back leg lowering towards the ground (but do not touch your knee to the ground). Your forward leg should bear most of the weight.

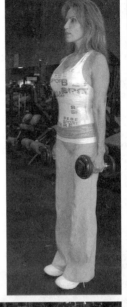

- Rise back up by pressing up through your front foot by driving your heel into the ground, and stand back up to original upright position. Repeat with the other leg. (Doing both legs is one rep).
- Keep your torso straight with your chest out, and your abs tight the entire time.
- Keep arms directly at your side throughout the movement.
- Inhale as you step forward and lower yourself. Exhale as you push yourself back up.

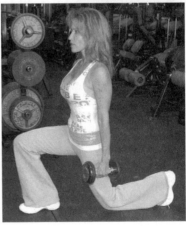

The "Do Nots"

- Lean over at the waist (or round out your back) while doing this exercise.
- Step forward too far as to stretch groin and hip area too much.
- Allow your arms and the dumbbells to swing.
- Push back up by pushing with the front foot allowing the heels to rise.
- Don't let your front knee go past your toes.

Exercise

Leg Extensions (Quadriceps)

- Sit up straight or lean back against the pad. Grasp the handles by the seat.
- Keep your toes pointed *upward* throughout the entire movement.
- Keep buttocks down on the seat throughout each rep.
- Straighten your legs to contract thighs at the top of each repetition.
- Slowly and smoothly lower the weight back on each repetition.
- Exhale when lifting; inhale when lowering the weight.

The "Do Nots"

- Lift the back of your legs off the seat at anytime.
- Drop your toes forward and/or relax your feet and ankle joint.
- Swing the weight with excessive speed.

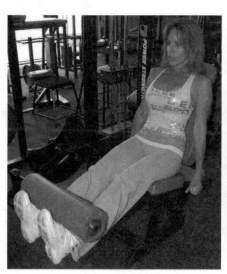 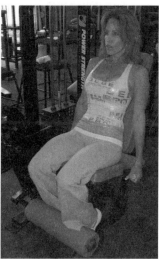

Leg Curls (Hamstrings)

- Lie face down on your belly, and position your feet on the machine with the back of your heels against the pad.
- Pin your hips down and curl the weight towards your back, pulling it up with the back of your heels (against the pad).
- Keep a tight hand grip so as to keep your body still.
- Keep your toes pointed up towards your shins the entire time.
- Contract your hamstrings at the top of the movement.
- Lower the weight slowly and smoothly.
- Exhale as you curl the weight up; inhale as you let it down.

The "Do Nots"

- Lift your hips upward.
- Turn your head side to side.
- Allow your pelvis to shift side to side.

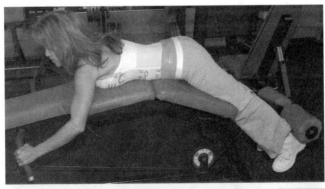

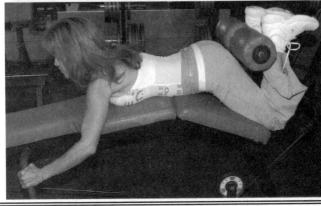

Standing Calf Raises (Legs: Calves)

- Position your feet shoulder width apart on the machine.
- Place your shoulders under the pads of the machine.
- While keeping your knees *slightly bent* and your back straight, stand up on your tippy toes on the front platform and focus on contracting your calf muscles.
- Lower slowly to a full comfortable stretch by bringing your heels towards the ground, then push back up, performing smooth controlled repetitions.
- Exhale as you push the weight up; inhale as you lower it.

The "Do Nots"
- Bounce up and down forcefully.
- Perform half-reps (get the full stretch at the bottom and extend all the way at the top).
- Allow your hips to move forward.
- Lean over from the waist.

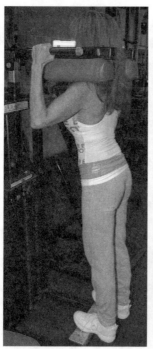 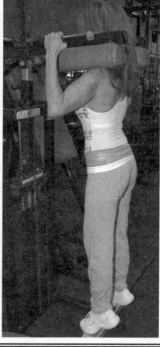

Seated Calf Raises (Legs: Calves)

- Sit in the calf machine with your back straight and feet *slightly closer* than a shoulder width apart.
- Place the balls of your feet on the machine
- Lift your heels as high as possible and contract the calf, then lower slowly as to get a full stretch at the bottom bringing your heels towards the ground.
- **Tip:** Push towards the pinky toe.
- Exhale as you push the weight up; inhale as you lower it.

The "Do Nots"
- Allow your feet to slide off so you are on your toes only.
- Swing your body back and forth while performing the repetitions.
- Perform half-reps, allow for a full comfortable stretch at the bottom of each repetition.

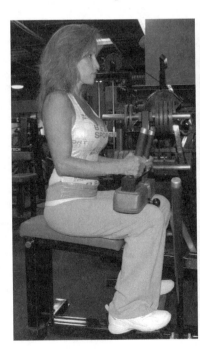 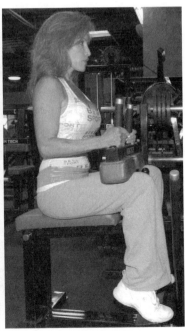

Crunches (Abdominals)

- Lie flat on your back on the floor.
- Bend your legs so the bottoms of your feet are touching the floor.
- Have your hands at the sides of your head resting <u>gently</u> behind your ears (not locked together).
- Keep your face parallel to the ceiling and your eyes looking straight up.
- Tighten your abs so your lower back is flat against the floor (at all times) and crunch your torso upwards, bringing your head up and forward.
- **Tip:** When crunching up, your neck, shoulders, head and arms should move <u>as</u> <u>one</u> <u>unit</u>. (Do not round your neck forward). Pretend there is a small ball under your chin at all times.
- Descend slowly always keeping constant tension on your abs, with *your back flat against the floor.*
- Exhale as you "crunch" upwards; inhale as you lower your body.

The "Do Nots"
- Never pull on the back of your head during the exercise.
- Jerk forward to perform a rep.
- Lift your feet off the floor during the exercise.
- Hold your breath during the exercise.
- Arch your lower back.

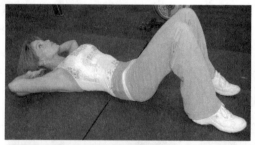

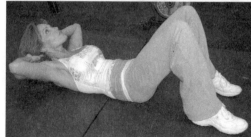

<u>Machine Pull-Downs to the Front</u> (Back)

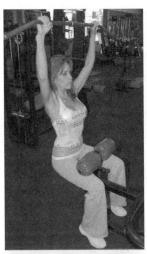

- Sit with your back straight in the seat and your feet flat on the floor.
- With an overhand grip, grab a standard pull-down bar about 4 to 6 inches wider than shoulder width.
- Using your hands as "hooks" and gripping the bar firmly (but lightly), pull the bar down towards the nape of your neck while simultaneously sticking your chest out (focusing on pulling your elbows straight down or slightly towards the back).

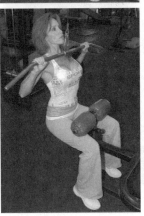

- Squeeze your shoulder blades together (pretend there is someone's finger on your upper spine, and you are pinching together your shoulder blades to touch it), and then allow the bar to slowly return up, keeping constant tension on your back muscles.
- Keep your thighs tucked under the machine pads fairly snug. This will create leverage for you during the movement.
- Exhale as you pull down; inhale as you release the bar back up.

The "Do Nots"
- Allow your chest to sink (concave) as you pull the bar towards the nape of the neck or upper chest.
- Allow your body to lift up and down out of the seat while performing your reps as this will take away your strength and leverage from the movement.
- Allow the bar to hit your chest or sternum with abrupt force.

Exercise

Machine or Barbell Press (Shoulders)

- Sitting on a machine or standing up, keep your back straight and your feet a little wider than shoulders. Look straight ahead.
- Hold the bar shoulder width with palms of hands facing forward.
- Push or "press" bar straight up until your arms are <u>almost</u> straight, but do not lock your elbows; then slowly lower the bar back down with the palms of your hands facing forward.
- Exhale as you press up; inhale as you lower.

The "Do Nots"
- Turn your head side to side or look up.
- Push up on your toes.
- Throw the weight up with your body.

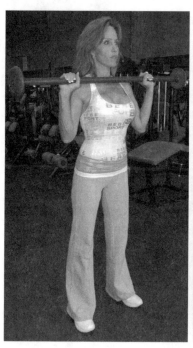 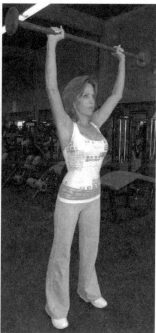

One-Arm Dumbbell Rows (Back)

- Place your right knee on a flat bench while your left leg is placed shoulder width apart on the floor and slightly bent.
- Lean over at the waist and place your right hand on the flat bench.
- Grab a dumbbell with your left hand with your palm facing the bench.
- While keeping your back straight, abs tight, chest slightly out, pull the dumbbell towards your waist (contracting your shoulder blade towards your spine) and lift your elbow above the level of your back.
- Lower the dumbbell slowly while keeping your back muscles and abs tight until your shoulder blade stretches back out away from your spine.
- After you do the number of reps indicated, switch sides (left knee on the bench, right leg on the floor) and do the same number of repetitions (this completes one set).
- **Tip:** Pretend your hands are "hooks" when you pull the weight up (don't grip the dumbbell too tightly).
- Exhale as you lift up; inhale as you lower the weight.

The "Do Nots"
- Overly rotate at the torso (or round your back).
- Turn your head from side to side.
- Sink your chest.
- Jerk the dumbbell up.

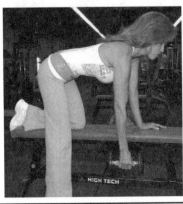 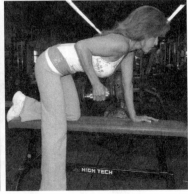

Exercise

Dumbbell Lateral Raises (Shoulders)

- Stand with your feet a little closer than shoulder width apart and your eyes looking straight ahead.
- Hold dumbbells directly at your sides and lift them away from the body, up until parallel with your shoulders. Keep your arms *slightly bent*.
- Keep a firm grip so the <u>backs</u> of your hands the entire time, face towards the ceiling with your pinky fingers higher than your index finger or thumb (like pouring a pitcher of milk).
- Lower the dumbbells slowly back to your sides.

The "Do Nots"
- Allow your body to swing in any direction.
- Allow your wrist to go limp, dropping dumbbells downward.
- Allow your elbow joint to straighten or "lock out".
- Turn your head from side to side.

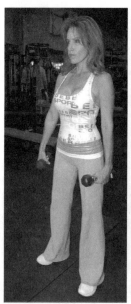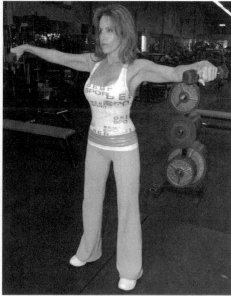

Stiff-Arm Pulldowns (Back)
- Stand in front of a lat pulldown or triceps pushdown cable machine.
- Use an overhand grip (palms away) and grab a straight triceps bar or lat pulldown bar about shoulder width apart.
- With your body slightly bent over at the waist and your back straight, keep your arms slightly bent and stationary, and push the bar down (with your back muscles doing the work) towards your thighs.
- Allow the bar to rise up slowly allowing for a nice stretch back to the top.
- Keep your chest out and your abs tight at all times.
- Keep your grip over the top of the bar at all times.
- Exhale as you push down; inhale as you re turn the bar back up.

The "Do Nots"
- Bring your heels off the ground.
- Bend your arms too much or completely lock your elbow.
- Sink your chest (round the back) at any time.
- Let your wrists or grip move.

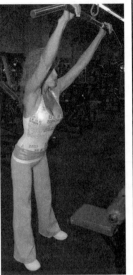

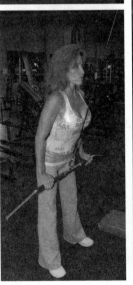

Reverse and Cross Crunches (Abdominals)
(See Workout 1)

Exercise

Unless noted, the exercises will be done the same as described in the previous *Exercise Descriptions and Instructions* section (these will be notated as "same exercise described").

Lunges (Legs)

Same as the exercise described. Use dumbbells. If you're traveling, do the exercises without them, but do more repetitions so each leg "feels it." For extra legwork, include two sets of *Step Ups* with or without dumbbells.

Push Ups (Chest)

Do standard (on toes) or on your knees (easier). Keep your hands flat on the floor slightly wider than shoulder width. Keep your back straight with pelvis slightly elevated and your abs tight. Your feet or knees should be placed hip width apart and balance on your toes. Lower your chest to the floor while always keeping a slight pinch together of your shoulder blades. Perform smooth movements with good rhythm. Lock out the arms at the top of the movement to also work tri-

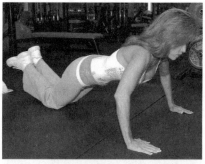
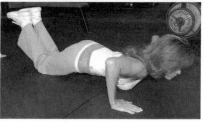

ceps. Do not sink (concave) your chest at anytime. Keep your chest protruding outward. Do not lower your pelvis or sag the lower back.

One-Arm Dumbbell Rows (Back)

Same exercise as described. *With resistance bands:* Place the middle of the band around a heavy object like a large table, bedpost or doorknob. Sit in a chair with your feet wider than shoulder width apart. Grab the handles of band and position them so the bands are stretched and tight, with your palms facing each other and your arms stretched out in front of you at chest level. Pull both hands towards your stomach while sticking your chest out and squeeze your shoulder blades together as you pull towards your abdominals. Stretch back to the beginning position, and then repeat. Use the same form, tips and "Do Nots" described in *One Arm Dumbbell Rows* (but you'll be doing it for both arms at same time).

Dumbbell Kickbacks or Band Extensions (Triceps)

With a dumbbell in each hand, standing, keeping a slight bend in the knees, keep your torso straight and your abs tight, and bend over at 45 degrees at the waist. Raise your elbows to your sides next to your ribs with your arms bent so the dumbbells are almost touching the front of your shoulders, and your palms facing your body. Keeping your elbows at your sides at all times, extend the dumbbells backwards and up towards the ceiling, locking out at the elbow to contract the triceps muscle. *With bands:* Stand on the bands, and perform the *Standing Bar Extension*, but do not bend 10-15 degrees at the waist (instead stand with your body straight). Your palms will be facing forward while holding the handles.

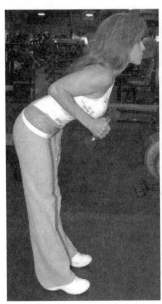 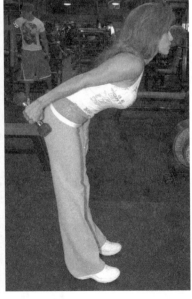

Exercise

Dumbbell Curls (Biceps)

Same exercise as described. *With bands:* Stand on the bands and follow the same instructions like you were using dumbbells.

Dumbbell Presses (Shoulders)

With dumbbells: Sitting on a chair, follow the same instructions for *Machine or Barbell Presses* (when holding dumbbells, your palms will face forward). *With bands:* stand on the bands, follow the instructions for the *Machine or Barbell Presses.* You'll be pressing the handles up over your head like dumbbells.

One Leg Standing Calf Raises (Calves)

Stand on either a stair or a phone book(s) that is high enough so your heel does not touch the ground at the bottom of the movement. Perform the *Standing Calf Raises*, but bend one leg back, so you are standing on (and supporting your body) with only one leg. Do all your repetitions on that leg and then do the other (both legs complete one set). If doing one leg is too hard, then stand normally and do both – just increase the repetitions and do as many as you can.

Crunches or Cross Crunches (Abdominals)

Same exercises as described.

These exercise instructions were provided with the assistance of Health Direct customer and personal trainer, Danny Kaczmarek. See his testimonial and picture on the first page of the next section.

The exercise model is *How to Completely Reshape Your Body* reader and *Health Direct* customer, Dawn. See her testimonial in *The Discovery* section.

References & Resources

"Top Southern California Trainer Shares Tips On Staying Lean And In-Shape Year-Round "

Danny has been a Certified Personal Trainer for over 15 years, is a Certified Micro-Current Therapist, and is just completing work to be a Doctor of Naturopathy.

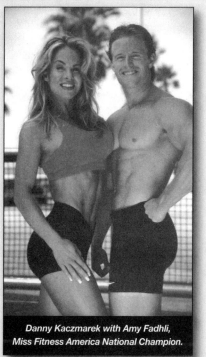

Danny follows a strict *Plan A* type regimen when "cutting" up (losing fat) and *Plan B* basics year-round, although he has always kept in above-average, excellent shape over the last ten-plus years I have known him.

Danny is also a firm believer in supplementation with correcting the digestive system and cleansing at the start of any health program – and considers it a *"major factor in staying healthy and vibrant."* Danny has recommended the supplements in this book to his clients over the last 10 years and comments:

Danny Kaczmarek with Amy Fadhli, Miss Fitness America National Champion.

"The first thing I notice with AminoSculpt is deeper, better sleep, and muscle hardening. I wake up more refreshed when using it and it really helps me lose those last layers of fat when I really want to trim down.

Sculpt n' Cleanse is easy to use and works great for slimming the waistline and eliminating toxicity. Also, Optimal Omega HP is the best Omega-3 fish oil available. I love the Astaxanthin in the product. Also, the product has no aftertaste, unlike other fish oil supplements. I notice it's easier to eat lower amounts of carbohydrates when I increase the dosage of these fish oils (sometimes up to 8-12 a day)."

Danny has a true passion for fitness, helping other people and the Lord's work – and is one of the best trainers in Southern California. You can learn more about Danny at: www.optimumtraining.net.

"Reference Materials and Resources For Starting Your Program Quickly"

This section is designed to provide quick and easy access to additional information referred to throughout this book.

Enclosed in this section, in the following order, are:

1. **How To Accurately Track Your Progress**

   Easy-to-use forms and information to assist you in *accurately tracking* your body reshaping and weight loss progress. This includes:

   • How to track your results
   • A form for measuring your body to chart your progress
   • A guide on how to use pictures to track your progress

2. **Where To Find The Products Mentioned In This Book, And Why I Recommend Them**

   Detailed information on why I recommend the supplements in this book, as well as a summary listing of all of them, and where to find them; and

3. **FREE Bonuses and Additional Information**

   Free Bonuses for my readers, as well as access to additional health information not included in this book.

   Make sure you fill out these forms and access the additional information when beginning your program.

"How To Accurately Track Your Results – Start By Throwing Your Scale Out..."

As you begin to reshape your body and lose fat, I want to clear up a common "myth," and instruct you on how to accurately track your progress.

There is a big difference between losing weight - and losing fat.

Although most people rely on their scale to tell them what is happening, it is a <u>highly</u> inaccurate <u>tool</u>. When you are losing weight the correct way, you will be *maintaining or gaining muscle, and losing fat.*

For example, what does the scale tell you when you lose 5 pounds of fat and gain 5 pounds of muscle? Answer – ZERO. So how do you tell what is happening?

<u>**Four Simple Ways**</u>:

1. **Inches** - measuring your body before you start and during your program.
2. **Clothing** - how they fit (when they become loose, baggy, etc. - see my before and after photos).
3. **Photos** - shows exactly how your body has changed!
4. **Bodyfat testing**

And if you cleanse know this: As you eliminate the build-up (dry fecal matter, mucus, etc.) - your weight may initially drop faster, level off, and then may slowly increase (because of lean muscle tissue).

DON'T WORRY OR BE CONCERNED ABOUT MUSCLE GAIN - it will *not* make your hips, thighs, or stomach larger. The muscle gain will be in your vital organs, and throughout your body where you need the muscle to support your body structure and its functions.

With men, the muscle gained will make you look more muscular and well-formed, especially if you are lifting weights. For women, if you lift weights (which I encourage you to do), you won't look muscular. Your body will look shapely, firm, toned and feminine - like when you were younger.

Bodyfat Testing...

An effective and easy way to monitor your bodyfat is by using is a skin caliper. Most local sports related doctors can do this for you - or maybe someone at your local gym. When I made my transformation I used skin calipers (*Note:* have the same person do it each time, at the same time of day, to help keep the measurements consistent).

Summary of Tracking Your Results...

To properly track your results:

1. Measure yourself every 2-3 weeks (see the form in this section to help you to do that).
2. Notice how your clothes are fitting (how many belt notches you use, etc.). Keep one set of "tight" clothes that are your starting benchmark.
3. Take before and after photos. You get used to seeing your body in the mirror every day, but when you look at these pictures - you will see the difference (there is a helpful guide for taking these later in this section).
4. If you want to (but not necessary), get your bodyfat checked.
5. You can weigh yourself when you begin - *but only again every 4 weeks - and don't worry if your weight goes up!*

Remember:
Gauge your progress by *how your clothes fit and your inches lost,* not your scale weight. This will help you achieve the body you really want.

Charting Your Progress

Use this form and the following tips to track the inches you are losing. The following instructions are tips and will tell you how to consistently do this.

- Note *where* you measured, so you can re-measure in the same place (measuring an inch or two away in a different spot will give you incorrect results).
- Always re-measure at the same time of day you took the previous measurement.

		Start	Week 3	Week 6	Week 9	Week 12
Date:						
Time:						
Neck:						
Chest:						
Waist:	*1) bellybutton*					
	2) waistline					
Arms:	*1) right*					
	2) left					
Hips:						
Forearms:	*1) right*					
	2) left					
Thighs:	*1) right*					
	2) left					
Calves:	*1) right*					
	2) left					

Tips on Measuring:

Neck: Measure straight around the middle of your neck.

Chest: Put the tape up to your underarms, like a tailor would, and measure straight around your back and chest (you can also take another measurement at nipple level).

Waist: 1) bellybutton - measure straight around from your belly button.
2) waistline – measure around your waistline

Arms: Measure the middle of your upper arm at its widest point.

Hips: Look sideways in a mirror and measure around the <u>widest</u> point of your hips.

Forearms: Measure a few inches down from the inner crease of your arm (opposite of elbow) at the widest point.

Thighs: Measure straight around the middle of your thigh at the widest point, usually around four inches up from the top of your knee cap.

Calves: Measure the calf muscle around the widest point.

Documenting your reshaping journey with *before*, *during*, and *after* photos is important as:

1. *You will see your results more accurately.* Photos are a good way to notice even subtle changes – especially when looking at your body from behind and the side.

2. *Your photos will inspire and motivate you to keep on your program and, once you achieve your ideal weight, to stay there, so you do not go back to how you looked before.*

3. And hey – let's face it – they are great to show people who thought you would not lose weight!

If taking photos is not that easy to arrange, just start your diet – do not delay it for any reason. If you do take photos, take them as soon as you can when you start.

Use the following tips to take the best possible photos:

1. **Positioning Your Body In The Photo:** Fill the photo as much as possible without cutting out any body parts. *Photographers:* get as close as you can to your subject.

2. **Film and Camera:** A digital camera is best. Polaroid cameras are not recommended. Disposable cameras are ok, but get close to your subject as these cameras tend to make things look further away.

3. **Outdoor Pictures:** For outdoor pictures, make sure the subject is facing the sun. The best light is in the early morning or the late evening when the sun is low. The next best light is on slightly cloudy days when your shadow is barely visible. Both of these prevent shadows and squinting eyes. Use the flash outdoors to brighten shadows.

4. **Background and Indoor pictures:** Avoid dark walls and rooms – these absorb the light from the flash. Be aware of what is behind you so you do not have trees and power poles sprouting from behind your head. Also, avoid having busy or complicated things behind you.

Who Is Health Direct And Why Do I Recommend These Products?

Unlike some authors, when I developed this program, and wrote and published the original version of this book, I didn't own – or even dream of owning – a nutritional supplement company. I do now – and it's a fascinating and inspiring story, so I'll explain it as it adds to the authenticity of this book and the obsession I have for improving the health and lives of others.

This program was originally researched and developed by me, for me, and without any intentions or plans of writing a book, or selling or developing products. As mentioned and elaborated on in the opening pages of this book and in *The Discovery* section, after years of trial and error and tens of thousand dollars spent on weight loss programs, books, supplements etc., I was still overweight and discouraged. Fortunately, I was also stubborn and didn't give up.

After all that *experience*, research, conferring with weight loss professionals, physicians, and pharmacists, I finally developed a "system" for my own use (which is contained in this book).

After quickly and safely losing weight, and dramatically reshaping my body (as seen in the pictures I took to track my progress), my friends and family noticed the results and wanted to do what I did. I scribbled some notes and coached them through it. They also got the same results – and their friends and family all wanted to do it too.

This wasn't my business or career; I was just a guy with a passion about health, who was excited to help other people achieve their dreams and desires of losing weight. Well, eventually it got overwhelming. Many people were calling, and I didn't have enough time to help them all (as there wasn't a book yet to explain it). I finally thought that I'd write a little 10 to 12 page "how and what to do" booklet for my family and friends. I figured this would free me of the calls.

As I was writing, I kept having these "they really need to know this and that" epiphanies. Also, I was anxious to share all the "insider" knowledge I had discovered about the weight loss industry, separating fact from fiction, and clarifying what was a realistic shape to achieve without drugs or a Hollywood "make-over job."

Well, 182 full-sized, 8½ x 11, pages later, I finally ran out of breath and ink, and had the original version of the *How to Completely Reshape Your Body* finished. But there was a problem...

How I Turned The Exorbitant Cost of Hard-to-Find Products Into Savings and Convenience for My Readers – And Eventually Into A Premier Line Of Cutting-Edge Premium Supplements...

The first problem I encountered was that the products I used – although high-quality, effective, and in my opinion, the best available at that time (that's why I used them) – were expensive and in some cases cost prohibitive ($90 for a 10 day supply of colon cleanser!).

The other problem was that the products were usually not available in stores. If people wanted to include any of them, they would need to go through a medical professional or nutritionist. In other words, they would have trouble finding and affording them.

A Creative Solution For My Readers...

After brainstorming with a close friend and business associate, we concluded that the best way was to buy the products I was recommending and have people call my office to get them. The concept was simple: *call one convenient location, get high-quality supplements at affordable prices (we reduced them to reasonable prices), and provide excellent customer service.*

Eventually another problem arose. As the demand for my book and clients grew, I couldn't control the quality or the supply of these products since they weren't mine. Also, I felt some could be better. I was uncomfortable recommending products that were not the best quality at all times – and that may not be readily available.

Health Direct Was Born

With the goal of providing the absolute best quality supplements, *Health Direct* was born. One-by-one, I made and/or got exclusives on the absolute best source of each product available. Also, I developed other products, which were not available, that I felt could assist some people to lose weight more efficiently, as well as improve underlying health challenges that prevent weight loss. Over the last 10 years it has grown into a complete line of premium weight loss, anti-aging, pain-relief, beauty, and general health products.

Why This Company Is Totally Different...

Here's the fun part about what I do and why Health Direct products really are different – and why I unconditionally guarantee them. Every Health Direct product has been developed for my personal use, and for the use of my family and friends. It never made sense to me to make a product that wasn't the best, sell it, and then use someone else's. So if I'm going to make it, I use it! It must be the absolute best available.

There are other good products available, but most other companies are selling products strictly as a "business to make money," so corners are cut and decisions are made to serve that end. *Not at Health Direct.* The products cost a little more because they are the absolute best available. And that's why when you use them, you'll see and notice a difference immediately. I unconditionally guarantee this or I will take back any product with no questions asked (call and ask the *Health Direct* Customer Service Department for details).

From Dead Broke To Over
One Million Customers Worldwide...

By the way, another interesting part of the story is that I was dead broke and deep in debt when all this happened. I borrowed $1,500 on my Mom's credit card to print the first books and to buy a small amount of the products I recommended. I operated out of a 575 square foot office, took calls, and processed and packed the orders myself.

I have even had a number of my original customers who came to work here at *Health Direct*, because of the life-changing results they experienced and their passion for health and assisting others. Since then, *Health Direct* has grown and the products have changed the lives of <u>over 1 million people worldwide</u>!

This "Lost" Weight Loss Secret Has Come Back To Life!

Over the years as *Health Direct* grew, my original book went out of print (after six printings). Most of our original customers still order because of how the insights they learned from the book have changed their health and bodies – as well as the continual results they get from the products.

In the last few years there's been a growing number of requests for this book! Just like when I first started, the noticeable results and great experiences my readers had and still have, have created this interest.

Also, in recent years, <u>I have been outraged by some of the misleading claims that various weight loss product sellers have made</u>, as well as the thousands of "new" weight loss books that promise the next greatest weight loss plans. But these plans completely miss the main reasons why people have trouble losing weight. Compound all that with <u>my dismay that many of these weight loss authors have never really been overweight, or done what they are promoting</u> (covered in detail in the opening pages of this book), and it was time for me to share my discovery again. I trust that this explains this...

Completely Revised And Turbocharged Edition With The Most Cutting-Edge Weight Loss And Health Information Available!

My original program and writings are still the same, and the ironic thing is, ten years later, the information and techniques not only remain valid, but many have been further substantiated by science!

I have revised the book, upgraded the information, and a made the program easier to understand and use. The valuable feedback from my previous readers assisted me greatly. Also, I have fine-tuned all the material and included some new, cutting-edge research, refinements, and supplements that will help you get even better and faster results than my original readers did!

Thank you for taking the time to invest in your health and for allowing me to share my discoveries with you. The remaining pages will show you where to get any products or materials referred to, and discussed in this book, as well as any special bonuses that may be available to you...

Product	Type	Details
Sculpt n' Cleanse	Colon Cleansing	See Pages (78-80)
AminoSculpt	Collagen Protein	See Pages (81-82)
Ready Fiber	Fiber and Prebiotic	See Pages (83-84)
Carb Cheater	Blood Sugar and Insulin Management	See Pages (85-86)
Nature's Optimal Nutrition	Complete Nutritional Support Multivitamin	See Pages (87-88)
Optimal Omega HP	Omega-3 Fish Oil	See Pages (89-90)
Binge Buster	Appetite and Craving Control	See Pages (91-92)
MSM	Pure Organic Sulfur Antioxidant	See Pages (93-94)
Premium Whey Protein Isolate	Pure Protein Shake (Meal Replacement)	See Pages (95-96)
Pure Inspiration	Pure Healthy Drinking Water	PureInspirationWater.com

To learn where to obtain any of these products, call 1-800-414-2064, Dept. 3000

Free Reader Bonuses

A s a reader of this book, you have qualified for special health bonuses – valued at hundreds of dollars – for FREE. This is a limited-time offer so please read this information and respond immediately.

When writing this book, my goal was to provide quickly accessible information so you could know what you wanted to do and start reshaping your body immediately. I could have easily written hundreds of additional pages on the topics of weight loss, body shaping and general health, but this additional information may not be needed by everyone, and would only slow down the process of you getting started.

Your Own Personal "Virtual Health Menu" and Resource

The solution I decided upon was *to continue to provide you* with additional and new information outside this book, in a customizable manner so that you can easily access what you want and when. In a way, it is your own health resource center.

Through a combination of my website, newsletters, and live tele-conferences, I can provide you with incredible health changing information that I continually research and receive on a daily basis.

I'm Even Letting You In My
Private "Inner Circle"

Over the years I have met some of the most amazing and prominent researchers, doctors, scientists, chemists, and medical professionals in the field of natural health. This format even lets me directly share information from these individuals, including some recent interviews I have done with the initial researcher and discoverer of Omega-3 fish oils; creator and patent holder of hydrolyzed collagen; and one of the foremost authorities on the use of powerful marine ocean-based nutrients for nutrition.

You'll Get All This For FREE

By simply registering below, you'll have access to all this information, plus:

- Special promotional money saving offers that become available from any suppliers I recommend.

- Delicious recipes you can easily and quickly make while on the eating program.

- Delicious protein-shake recipes that you can use as quick, convenient, and cost-saving meal replacements on the program.

- Additional exercises including instructions, and tips for burning fat and shaping your body.

- Advanced exercises for continually building a healthy, toned and active body.

- Tips and success stories from my other readers on how they are using the material in this book to successfully lose weight and improve their health.

- Exercise and nutritional instructions from some of the best personal trainers – that would normally cost you over $50-100 an hour to consult or train with.

- Continual updates on the newest scientific research developments, studies and findings. My network of contacts in the scientific, medical and nutrition field is extensive, and I'll pass all the breakthrough discoveries on to you!

- New supplement information that becomes available. You'll be the first to know about the most cutting-edge life enhancing nutrients and supplements available!

- Special "alumni" discounts on additional copies of this book, and on any future editions, as well as the other books and publications I author.

- Critiques, evaluations, and reviews of weight loss and other health supplements available.

- And much, more!

Yours FREE By Acting Now...

This is a limited-time offer, so please act now. Normally, there is a yearly subscription for this information, but as part of my 10-Year Anniversary Special, I am waiving the fee for the first 997 readers.

This Is A Limited-Time Offer –
Please Act Immediately

To receive access to all these special bonuses and information, simply:

1.   **Call toll-free: 1-800-414-2064, Dept. 3000**

2.   Go to: **www.reshapeforlife.com/bonuses.html**

3.   Or, fill out and mail in the certificate below...